The new Easy Exhaustion Cure
For Workaholics And Overachievers

By Elwin Robinson

Foreword by Sarma Melngailis

©2010, All Rights Reserved

ISBN-13: 978-1463740733
ISBN-10: 1463740735

Table Of Contents

Foreword by Sarma Melngailis — 6
Acknowledgements — 9

Introduction

Who Is This Program For? — 10
Why Create An Exhaustion Cure? — 13
Priorities — 15
Are You Exhausted? — 17
How Long Will It Take? — 22
Too Much Information — 24
Keeping It Doable — 26
The Importance of a Compelling Vision — 30
Program Outline — 33

Part One

Recharging Energy — 38

STEP 1
Taoist Tonic Herbs For The Kidneys — 39

STEP 2
Greens — 44
Green Foods — 46
Green Drinks — 52
Green Superfoods — 57

STEP 3

Minerals	64
Magnesium	70
Sodium	76
Potassium	82
Zinc	87
Manganese	91
Iodine	95
Selenium	99
Bonus Mineral: Silica	103

STEP 4

Supplements	107
Vitamin C	109
Daily Multiple	114
Pregnenolone	118

STEP 5

Habits	121
Grounding	123
Spring Water	130
Sleeping at the Right Time	136
Eating Early	139
Breathing Clean, Fresh Air	141
Relax	144
Bonus Habit: Breathing Exercises	148
A New Approach to Energy	156

Part Two
Storing Energy — 159

STEP 1
Astringent Tonic Herb: Schizandra — 161

STEP 2
Essential Fats — 164
Omega 3 Fats — 167
Omega 6 Fats — 174

Part Three
Spending Energy Wisely — 178
Taoist Tonic Herbs For The Heart — 181

Bonus Section
Ideally Don't — 188
The Dilemma — 191
Stimulants — 193
Sugar — 197
Cooked Fat — 201
High Protein Diets — 204
Processed Foods — 207
Sleep Deprivation — 210

Final Thoughts
Keep It Simple	215
Get Leverage	216
Reassess Your Health	220

Additional Information And Resources
Shopping List	226
Daily Schedule	228
Starting Dosage	228
Intermediate Dosage	232
Full Dosage	236
Maintenance Dosage	241
Additional Dietary Recommendations	245
Additional Supplement Recommendations	247
Additional Practice Recommendations	249
Information Resources	251
Product Resources	254
About Lion Heart Solutions	257

Foreword

Being tired now and then is something most people are familiar with. But what happens when it's day after day, and you start to feel like it's not just temporary? When you sleep for hours, and you're still tired? You drink your usual coffee (or raw cacao drink, or whatever) and it's not giving you the buzz it used to.

You know you should exercise, do yoga, relax, ease your workload, but sometimes those things literally aren't possible. In my case, I also felt I was eating the healthiest food possible – fresh, organic, vegan raw food, including loads of greens – and yet still every day I felt… tired.

By the time I found Elwin, I was not just exhausted to the core. I was also fully confused and frustrated, with a good dose of shame. I was frustrated that no-one seemed to understand, and frustrated at getting too much obvious advice that I already know but can't exactly follow, because I'm literally too busy.

Meanwhile, I knew it was only getting worse, and that even if it were possible to take a vacation, a week wouldn't fix me. I felt as if I would need months of drooling in a hammock before I might begin to feel rested.

What is wrong with me? I'm not supposed to not feel good. I've written two books on raw food in which I describe the vibrant energy and amazing wellness eating this way brings about. But I don't always follow my own advice.

And because I have my own business which is still in its early stages, I live in a way that leaves me confused when someone asks me, "What do you do in your spare time?" or my favourite, "Let's get together when you're not busy." Spare time? Not busy? What does that mean??

It was online that I found Elwin. Or, he found me. He'd read some of my rants online, my sometimes very TMI Twitter/Facebook posts, and made a comment that initially made me angry. This was a response to an angry tweet of mine where he suggested perhaps I was angry because my liver wasn't functioning properly. What?? (That's exactly how I replied to his comment, except in all caps... WHAT?!?).

Then I was thinking, I have to look up who this guy is. He's probably one of those spaced out always-happy people that I simultaneously envy and want to punch. I started fishing around his website and watching his videos and realized, wow. This guy seems to know what he's talking about. Because he's been there.

I wrote to him and thus began my long distance affair in healing with Elwin. We spoke on the phone for two hours during which time he asked a ton of questions. I immediately felt comfortable, like I could tell him anything. He explained so much to me in that first phone call.

Finally, for the first time I felt real hope, and even excitement. Here's someone who understood, was completely non-judgmental, and explained everything in a way I could completely understand and relate to. And best of all, I wasn't left having to commit to something I couldn't commit to.

In the past, I'd say, yes, I'll do this or that meditation, I'll listen to these CDs daily for 20 minutes, I'll start every day with a routine of yoga exercises, I'll gaze at the sun, I'll show up every week for acupuncture, healing work, etc. I'll rest, I'll love myself more, whatever.

But then these things have always been mostly unrealistic for me, given what I do, where I am, and how I live, right now, which isn't changing any time soon. So I need something I can actually do. Elwin understands this!

I hope he and this program helps you as much as it's helped me. Thank you, Elwin.

Sarma Melngailis

Founder and Executive Chef at Pure Food and Wine, the world's top Raw Food Restaurant; author of Living Raw Food and Raw Food Real World and President of oneluckyduck.com

Acknowledgements

This book wouldn't have been possible without the help and support of many people, far too many to list.

Thank you to everyone who showed me by example what to do, as well as what not to do.

Thank you to Sarma Melngailis for inspiring me to create this program, and to Kerenza and Lee Turner for supporting me all the way. You're the best!

Thank you to Joe Best for introducing me to the possibilities of the internet and encouraging me, to Sarah Best of Get Fresh magazine for helping me realise I was born to write, and to Shazzie for your incredibly valuable support.

Thank you to Lewis, Adrian and Paul, who all contributed, and without whom this program wouldn't have been possible.

Thank you so much to all of you. My love and appreciation for you is boundless.

And much love and thanks to all my past, present and future clients for making me aware of how necessary this program is: you're the reason I do this.

I dedicate this program to all those who've had enough of struggling and making do, who want to experience life fully and have an abundance of energy to do it. Your solution starts here:

Introduction
WHO IS THIS PROGRAM FOR?

This program has been created especially for those people who are busy, stressed, working really hard, usually with the best of intentions, and who end up exhausted as a result.

I created this program after coming to realise, through my own experience as well as working with clients and communicating with people from all walks of life, that no one was providing people in this position with any real solutions.

How do I define 'real solutions?'

Approaches that are truly actionable despite the fact that you may already be: busy, stressed and exhausted.

Anyone who is in this position knows that dedicating lots of time and energy to improving your health and increasing your energy levels tends to feel like a total impossibility.

So I had to come up with something that is *easy*:

  Easy to understand

  Easy to implement

  Easy to follow through on

Does this mean that this program is only of use to you if you're busy, hard working, and already very stressed and deeply exhausted?

Do you need to be a workaholic or overachiever to get some benefit?

The answer is a resounding:

ABSOLUTELY NOT!

This program will benefit you no matter who you are, no matter what you do and no matter where you come from.

The only limiting factor could be your ability or willingness to buy the needed resources, as outlined in this course. This is really a matter of priorities though, if you make your health your number one priority, you will find a way!

Most people don't make their health their priority, which is why most people don't invest in their health until they have a health crisis, when it can often seem too late.

However, if you want to pre-empt a health crisis, and steer your life in the direction of radiant health and abundant energy NOW, rather than later, or if you'd like to encourage others you care about to do the same, this program is a perfect starting place.

If, however, your exhaustion is caused by major factors like weak immunity, high toxicity, metabolic or hormonal problems, or other serious conditions, rather than simply overwork and stress, I can't guarantee that following this program alone will CURE your exhaustion.

It will, undoubtedly, improve your situation and it may resolve it, but other approaches may need to be taken as well as the approaches outlined here.

Please see the resource section at the back of this book for people and places that can provide more useful information.

Remember that no matter how bad things may have become that there is always a way, if you are determined enough. If you are still lost as to how to proceed if you have a serious condition, please do feel free to contact me and I'll provide a complete program for you if I can, or refer you to someone who can help in the unlikely event that I can't.

However, whatever else you do, whoever else you see, I promise you that the recommendations in this program will always be helpful as a foundation. So follow through on them all consistently, and you may be surprised to find you'll improve to an almost miraculous degree over time.

Why Create An Exhaustion Cure?

Stress and exhaustion always go hand in hand. In fact stress, when unresolved, inevitably leads to exhaustion. Exhaustion in turn can lead to a whole host of other health problems.

I created this program for all those who are low on energy, who've realised it, who've had enough, and who now just need to be told what to actually do to make it better.

I created it initially for myself, when I realised, with some frustration, that no-one else was offering any real solutions.

I created it because I was tired of constantly making compromises with myself because I lacked the energy to follow through on what I knew was the right thing to do.

I created it because I was tired of feeling helpless and weak, like everything was just too much for me, like I couldn't do the simplest thing without feeling overwhelmed.

I created it because I was tired: tired of being a slave to addictions and cravings, tired of feeling like I wasn't in charge of my own behaviour.

Basically, I created it because I felt like I had no choice. And I'm so glad I did. Now I get to not only feel great and have an abundance of energy, I get to share this knowledge with other people, who consequently feel great and do the same, so that a ripple of abundant energy becomes a tidal wave of health!

Now, after extensive refining, practice, testing and experience, you have in your hands the complete program which guarantees the same results for you if you apply the steps persistently.

This is for all of you who know you have a greater destiny, a purpose in life, whether you know what it is yet or not.

This is for all of you who realise that all that's really holding you back is a lack of energy, the energy to be clear on what you're doing, the energy to follow through on your true purpose in life, and the energy to keep following through until you get there.

This is for all of you who realise that suffering and depletion is an unnatural state, a warning signal telling you something is wrong, not a way of life.

When you're no longer exhausted, when you have an abundance of sustainable energy and deep reserves of core energy, everything becomes clearer and easier to understand; everything flows and starts to fall in to place effortlessly.

Even more importantly, you start to feel great most of the time as your dominant emotional states go from: fear, anger, worry, stress and anxiety, to: gratitude, love, curiosity and a sense of renewed awe and wonder for life's abundance.

The astonishingly great news you'll soon experience for yourself is this:

It's all just an upgrade of energy away!

Priorities

There are three levels of priority for the recommendations contained in this program, indicated by three 'awards':

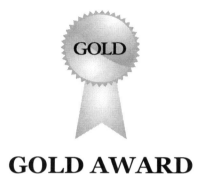

GOLD AWARD

These gold awards are **top priority**, and implementing them as part of your daily routine is essential for guaranteed results. Of course you will still make improvements leaving out some of these top priority steps, but for a simple, easy and total cure to exhaustion all these steps need to be followed.

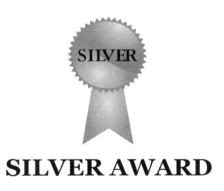

SILVER AWARD

All the steps in this category are **highly recommended**, but may not be possible, and are not absolutely essential. Success on the program does not depend on these steps, but is considerably helped by implementing them.

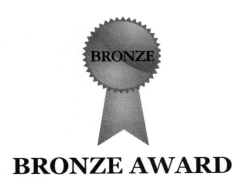

BRONZE AWARD

Ideally implement these steps too, but they're often difficult for some people to do, so they can be ignored or left until you are further along in the program, when you have more energy and are ready for these more challenging steps.

If you do follow *all* the recommendations made in every step of this program, GOLD, SILVER and BRONZE, your progress is likely to be truly extraordinary

Are You Exhausted?

It can be very useful and enlightening to complete a questionnaire to assess where you're at now. It's also great to have a guide to compare and thereby quantify your progress once you've been on the program for a month, two months, three months and beyond.

There's another questionnaire at the end of the program you can use to assess your progress.

The Easy Exhaustion Cure Questionnaire

Score the questionnaire as follows:

0 for rarely or never

1 for sometimes

2 for frequently or always

1. Do you still feel tired 30 minutes after waking up?

2. Do you need a stimulant like tea, coffee or a cigarette to get started in the morning?

3. Do you need a stimulant like tea, coffee or a cigarette to keep you going throughout the day?

4. Do you crave sweet foods?

5. Do you crave starchy foods like bread, pasta, potatoes and crisps?

6. Do you feel like you need an alcoholic drink by the end of the day?

7. Are you overweight and do you have great trouble losing weight, despite dieting?

8. Do you have frequent slumps of energy?

9. Do they happen especially after meals?

10. Do you have mood swings?

11. Do you have difficulty concentrating?

12. Do you struggle to get out of bed in the morning?

13. Do you use the snooze button on your alarm in the morning?

14. Does your memory fail you for things which you consider important?

15. Does your sex drive feel lower than it was?

16. Do you tend to get overwhelmed easily?

17. Do you find it a struggle to adapt to changes in circumstances in life?

18. Does life seem to be moving too fast?

19. Do you feel your life is frequently immersed in some kind of drama?

20. Do you get dizzy, tired or irritable if you go for longer than 5 hours without eating something or taking a stimulant like tea, coffee or a cigarette?

21. Do you feel like you're ageing prematurely?

22. Do you frequently feel frustrated?

23. Do you frequently feel tired throughout the day?

24. Do you feel like no matter what you do it's never enough?

25. Have you had more than two colds or infections in the last two years?

26. Do you have dark circles under your eyes?

27. Do you feel more tired after exercise or exertion?

28. Do infections tend to linger?

29. Do you suffer from any inflammatory conditions like eczema or asthma?

30. Do you have any fungal conditions?

31. Do you become anxious easily?

32. Do you find yourself getting angry or annoyed over little things?

33. Do you feel a lack of motivation?

34. Do you have problems getting to sleep?

35. Do you have problems staying asleep?

Add up your total score _____ out of 70

What your score means:

- *If you scored between 0 and 10:*

FULL TANK

Congratulations, you are already fairly or even very healthy. I would suspect that either you've already done some work on your health, or you're fairly young, or you're one of the lucky few who naturally have an abundance of reserve energy. You will still benefit from any or all of the parts of this program you decide to implement.

- *If you scored between 11 and 30:*

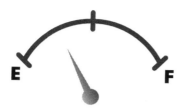

TIME FOR A REFILL

You will definitely benefit from doing this program, and would be well advised to do all the Gold Award priority steps, as well as doing as many as possible of the Silver and Bronze Award priority steps. A complete recovery is definitely possible by following the steps of this program consistently.

- *If you scored over 30*

RUNNING ON EMPTY

You will definitely benefit from following all the steps in this program that you can. A complete cure of your exhaustion may involve additional guidance; please check the 'Resources' section at the end of this book. Your recovery may take longer than a few months, but I promise you with the additional steps that I may advise if you contact me, and with persistence, you will make a full and complete recovery.

How Long Will It Take?

For everything I'm going to recommend to you throughout the course of this program, you're going to get significant results if you follow through for **90 days.**

If you follow through for **30 days** and you do all the steps recommended every day, or at least six days a week, you're going to experience an improvement in your health.

If you do the steps recommended for three months you're going to experience a significant improvement in your health and energy levels; and, if you do the steps for **a whole year**, you're going to experience a total transformation in your health to the point where you *won't even recognise who you were when you started the program.*

Now, I know a year can seem like an insufferably long time. Despite all the quick fixes and magic bullets that are being sold out there, the reality is this:

Real recovery from chronic exhaustion, which has taken years and often decades to build up, doesn't happen overnight.

This is the Easy Exhaustion Cure, not the Immediate Exhaustion Cure, simply because it's not possible to cure an energy depletion state immediately. You can get a jump start, and in fact that's exactly what following the steps in this program will give you, but, to continue the car analogy, you still need to continue to recharge your batteries for a while afterwards.

There's no getting around this. What you can do is make the process as effortless, painless and enjoyable as possible. That's what this program is for.

Suppressing the symptoms for a little while is easy. And that's what almost everyone else will offer you – symptom suppressors – despite the fact they may claim to 'cure' you. You're probably here because you've already discovered that they don't really work.

If you really think about it though, the fact that, with this program, you can make up for twenty or thirty or forty or fifty or more years of exhaustion within the space of a year is actually truly incredible, and the fact you can feel significantly better within 90 days is amazing.

Of course your recovery rate will depend partly on where you're starting from, indicated by your score on the questionnaire, and partly on whether you incorporate all the steps I've mentioned, or only the top priority ones.

Should you continue the steps described after you've finished the program? Ideally yes. With the few exceptions noted in the text, a lot of these steps are highly beneficial to you all the time – they're just crucial when you're exhausted.

Too Much Information

This program is about curing your exhausted state once and for all. It's not here to teach you about biochemistry, nutrition, herbalism, food, agriculture, environmentalism, physiology or any other academic subject. You'll only learn the bare minimum you need to know to get results. This program is created for busy people. For that you'll be taught step by step:

- **What to consume or do**
- **Why to do it (very briefly)**
- **How to do it**
- **How long to do it for**
- **How much to do or take**
- **What to buy (if applicable)**
- **Where to buy from (in the Resources section)**
- **Any warnings**

Every recommended step will have a:

Description
What it is, and why you should do it

Recommended Form
Best form to use, if applicable

Recommended Dosage
A recommendation as to amounts, frequency and duration

Action Step
Something to do right now!

Caution
Any relevant warnings. Although everything in this program is extremely safe, it is possible to have too much of a good thing, including oxygen and water. The Taoists teach moderation and balance in everything. Ignore at your own risk!

If you are interested in finding out more information about the scientific evidence, long history of use, traditional usages, anecdotes, testimonials and many benefits of the products and practices recommended herein, please refer to the Information Resources chapter at the end of this book.

This program will focus exclusively on you getting results. If at any point you feel overwhelmed or uninterested by the information provided during the **Description**, please just skip directly to the **Action Step** and **Recommended Dosage** section of each chapter, whilst checking the cautions, and go for it!

The program is designed so that you never need to know what these things are or why you're taking or doing them, if you're uninterested, or if you don't have the time or energy to learn about them.

All you really need to know is:

I did the **Action Step**, at the **Recommended Dosage**, heeding any **Cautions**, and **It Worked**.

When you're no longer exhausted you may have more time, energy and inclination to find out how they worked, and why they worked.

Keeping It Doable

In order to keep the program simple you're only going to be focusing on and working with three different areas of life, which are unavoidable anyway, no matter how exhausted you may already be:

You're going to be looking at improving:

    1. What you eat

    2. What you drink

    3. How you rest

That's it.

Notice I say *how* you rest, not how *long* you rest *for*. I realise there's a possibility that you only have the option of sleeping six hours a night, or maybe four hours a night or even less.

Perhaps you've just had a baby, or you have an unavoidable deadline at work. You're not going to be excluded from getting results in this program just because you're not able to get the amount of rest which people generally say is ideal.

But, you are going to be excluded from the results of this program if you don't follow the advice on *how* to rest, so that's a really crucial distinction I want you to take note of.

Notice also that there are a lot of things I didn't include. I didn't include exercise, I didn't include mental attitude, in fact I didn't include a lot of things which a lot of other people insist on, not because I think they're irrelevant, but because someone who is already exhausted is already overwhelmed, and understandably unwilling to take on new activities.

But what you're already going to be doing, because it's unavoidable, is: you're already going to be eating, you're already going to be drinking and you're already going to be sleeping, even if it's not very much.

So we're just going to look together at the three areas of life that you're already doing anyway, which you have to do as a default, and we're going to look at turning those around, mainly by adding things into your life.

Near the end of the program I'm going to suggest a few things which it would be *ideal* to remove from your life, but we're going to look primarily at that which we're going to add to your life.

Everything that I'm later going to suggest you remove from your life is going to be optional because, let's face it, when you're exhausted or overwhelmed, the idea of removing anything which seems to keep you sane, which seems to keep you balanced or which seems to keep your energy levels up, is going to be unthinkable!

So, rest assured, I'm not going to ask you to stop doing anything which, as far as you're concerned, is keeping you going. During the program I'm just going to ask you to add things into your life, which are going to be a better alternative to some of those things that you've been using to keep you going.

Eventually, if you stick at the program, those things that I recommend you ideally avoid will have less of an appeal to you anyway, simply because you won't need them anymore. You don't need coping mechanisms when you're thriving, only when you're struggling.

The problem is, when you try to force yourself not to have these coping mechanisms, this ultimately always creates an internal conflict. This is where you're fighting yourself, saying something like: 'I shouldn't do this but I really want to.'

Creating internal conflict is a drain of energy, more than anything else. Therefore during the duration of this program you need to avoid these at all costs.

Absolutely nothing recommended in this program should create internal conflict inside you. If you decide you really can't do what I recommend, then you simply don't do it. That's it. No self-punishment, guilt or recriminations. Just make an honest decision and stick to it. If you change your mind, implement your new decision and stick to that.

This simple mental attitude I just described will save you vast quantities of energy if you apply it, and has the added bonus of filling you with a feeling of true self esteem. This feeling is probably the most undervalued feeling ever, and the feeling that all addictions and cravings are merely an unsatisfying substitute for.

If you decide that *you really* can't give anything up which I recommend in the '**Ideally Don't**' chapter that perhaps you'd ideally like to give up, then don't give them up! Be absolutely happy with the fact you've made a decision and stuck to it. Only you know your own capacities.

Do not under any circumstances create any more internal conflicts inside yourself. Do what I recommend, or if you're not going to do it then don't do it. Whatever you do though, don't feel like you *should* have and get lost in shame or guilt. These feelings really will do more harm than any of the things that you're recommended to avoid.

The Importance Of A Compelling Vision

Extensive research has proven, beyond any doubt, that those people who set a *written goal* for what they want to achieve, who have a definite plan for fulfilling that goal (that's what you've got here, The Easy Exhaustion Cure), and who frequently imagine themselves already having fulfilled that goal, are massively more likely to succeed at that goal, more quickly and more easily.

So what are your goals around energy and exhaustion?

A lot of times people think in 'moving away from' values, like "I don't want to be tired all the time" or "I don't want to wake up feeling like I want to go back to sleep for another year anymore."

It's fine if your mind operates this way, but just as a mental exercise, how about spending a few minutes now just attempting to reframe you desires in the positive?

So for example "I don't want to be tired anymore" might become "I want to have an abundance of energy". Or 'I don't want to wake up feeling like death warmed up" might become "I want to be filled with a joyful enthusiasm for life from the moment I wake up." See how this process works? It's a technique which is called *reframing*, and it's one of the most important mental techniques you'll ever learn, if you choose to use and apply it.

Just spend a few minutes now thinking about your goals around exhaustion and energy. When you've come up with a few, at least two, write them in this box, or somewhere else where you'll remember where they are:

MY GOALS

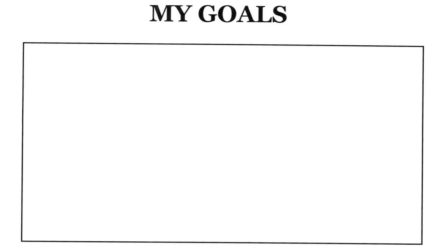

Now here's the most important bit of all: imagine yourself already having achieved these goals. See yourself radiating vitality. Feel yourself buzzing with energy. Imagine how you'll feel, what you'll do, where you'll go.

Imagine yourself doing all the things you've put off because you had no energy. Imagine what you'll be able to create, to produce, to achieve, to learn, to discover. Imagine who you'll have the energy to fully connect with, and what you'll have the energy to do.

Build a really compelling image, in your imagination, of the person you're going to become as a result of doing this program, and imagine it's already happened.

If you do this every day, first thing in the morning and/or last thing at night, in combination with the other, more practical steps in this program, I guarantee you you'll be absolutely shocked at how quickly and dramatically you reach your goals.

Warning: Only do this if you really want to get better. If you in any way enjoy being exhausted and weak and the sympathy and support you believe it engenders, this technique is extremely dangerous!

Program Outline

This program is divided into three fundamental steps:

1. You need to RECHARGE your energy

2. You need to STORE your energy

3. You need to CONSERVE your energy

In order to recover from exhaustion long-term you of course need to recharge your energy reserves. This is an absolutely crucial part of recovery from exhaustion.

However you can't just leave it there, that's only the first step. You also need to retrain your body to store your reserve energy efficiently, and you need to stop using up more than you can spare. It sounds quite obvious when you hear it, right?

But I've never found anyone, anywhere, outside of Taoist Medicine, who emphasises the importance of all three steps, or who teaches you how to do it. That's why this program was created.

This three-step model can be applied to many areas of life. It compares very closely with recovering effectively from a negative financial situation, like debt, where the resource you're lacking isn't life energy, but money.

If you're broke, you need more money, right? But that's only the start. You also need to save and invest that money sensibly, and spend it with a little vigilance and restraint. Only then can you have an abundance of wealth.

Lottery winners often illustrate this point well when, within a few years of winning a huge lottery jackpot, they usually end up where they started financially, or often even worse off. They did the first step, they got more money, but they never learned to store it effectively, or spend it carefully. Before long they're broke again.

As with money, so with energy. We need to do all three steps to have an abundance of energy.

We need to:

    1. Get more Energy

    2. Save it wisely and

    3. Spend it sensibly

It's very common, especially for those of us brought up with a western mindset, to always be very focused on getting *more*. It's what we're being told to focus on all the time by advertising, it's what everyone around us is focused on, so it's constantly being reinforced within us. We feel we need more energy, we need more money, we need more time, we need more attention and we need more stuff!

Unfortunately though, just getting more energy isn't enough. Just like with money, it doesn't matter how much you're earning – if you're spending more than you're earning, then at the end of the year you're still going to have a deficit: you'll have less money than you started with, and, if you're like the vast majority of people, then you'll actually have less than nothing – you'll be in debt. This is true for any economy, whether of money or energy.

This debt situation is in fact precisely what happens too within your body, as the adrenals borrow Reserve Energy, known in Traditional Taoist Medicine as Jing, from the kidney organ system, just to keep you going. This energy is like our 'emergency savings' and when we don't replenish those savings at the next available opportunity (which is exactly what I'm going to show you how to do with this program), we're potentially in serious trouble health and energy wise.

This state of energy depletion is actually more serious than any debt because at least with financial debt there's a do-over clause: it's called bankruptcy. The penalty for total energy depletion is more severe – it's called death!

The only form of 'do-over clause' when it comes to energy is known as reincarnation, not a strategy that I'd like to rely on. But don't panic, you're not bankrupt in energy yet, or you wouldn't be capable of reading this. And it's never too late to turn it all around and become an energy 'millionaire'.

When this state of energetic depletion does occur, we tend to get edgy, anxious and worried – often without realising why – and we soothe ourselves, often with distractions or numbing agents, to alleviate our anxiety, which of course make the problem worse!

All the negative effects noted by sociologists caused by financial deprivation on the individual also apply to those suffering from a lack of reserve energy, and they are magnified tenfold.

You start to sense on a deep level that your energy reserves are low and this understandably worries and stresses you. Worry and stress make the situation worse as they are a massive drain on reserve energy, and this is a downward spiral that many people tragically never escape from.

For more information on how this situation comes about please refer to the bonus audio '**Overcoming Exhaustion**' that comes with this program.

Enough of explaining the problem. There's an excellent quote by a brilliant man called Anthony Robbins that says "Spend 10% of the time focusing on the problem, and 90% of the time focusing on the solution."

That's what you're going to be doing from now on, for the rest of this program, and for the next 90 days *at least*: focusing on what's important – the solution – which is, one more time:

1. **Get more Energy**

2. **Save it wisely** and

3. **Spend it sensibly**

PART ONE

Recharging Energy

This first part of this program, **Recharging Energy**, is the most crucial to get right.

It's been highlighted that you need to realise it's not the only step, because it's important to realise there are more steps. But really, the second and third steps are actually very easy to implement if you've done the first step; the second and third steps being **Storing Energy** and **Conserving Energy** respectively.

The only problem most people have with the second and third step is they don't realise they exist, or they don't know what to do. Doing them is actually very straightforward.

However, **Recharging Energy** is going to be your primary area of focus throughout this program, as there are quite a few parts to implement in your life to really do it well.

They all boil down to: FIVE SIMPLE STEPS

There are five simple steps in this program to Recharge your Energy. They are:

Taoist Tonic Herbs: Kidney Tonics

Greens

Minerals

Supplements

Habits

STEP 1
TAOIST TONIC HERBS FOR THE KIDNEYS

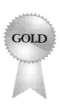

Description

Taoist tonic herbs are incredible. You will always remember the time you first discovered them.

Kidney Tonic Herbs will help you to replenish your energy on a really deep level, because, like I explain in depth in the 'Overcoming Exhaustion' bonus interview, the kidneys are where the body stores its reserve energy.

Therefore, you want to increase the strength of your kidney organs as a top priority. When they are tonified, which basically means strengthened, they will be able to store your reserve energy more efficiently and the recharging as a result of the other four steps will be effortless and easy.

They help to recharge your energy because as soon as your kidneys are stronger, every cell of your body will be able to hold more energy.

These tonic herbs are also particularly excellent for

dehydration. Obviously drinking water is vital too, but often for exhausted people, no matter how much water they drink, they still feel thirsty. These herbs are excellent for this.

In fact, the particular blend of herbs recommended here makes an excellent sports drink, as it's so hydrating. Anyone who is exhausted, stressed or anxious is dehydrated, no matter how much they may drink.

Dehydration, stress and exhaustion go hand in hand, and rehydrating is an absolutely essential step in curing exhaustion, as well as anxiety and stress. We'll look at that more closely when we discuss water.

The Taoist tonic herbs particularly recommended for exhaustion are:

Shizandra

Ho She Wu, also called Polygonum

Prepared Rehmannia

Ligustrum

Dioscorea

Glehnia

Achyranthes Root

Now that you have this list, what you need to do is find these particular herbs, or more ideally a herbal blend, either a tea blend or tablets, that contain most if not all of these herbs. Then, you need to make sure you consume them, consistently, **every day** throughout the course of this program.

Recommended Form

You can brew the whole herbs in water and prepare as a tea, drinking hot or cold, straight away or later on. The tea can be kept fresh in the fridge for a considerable period of time, up to a week. Lion Heart Herbs' Rejuvenate, which I formulated, is an excellent choice.

It's also possible to buy them and consume them in tablet form as an extract. Make sure they are an extract if you get them in tablets, otherwise they'll be a waste of time. You'd have to take dozens of tablets a day to get any useful effect, and many herbs have to be extracted in some way to be of benefit.

There are many other forms of these herbs, but these two forms are the most common ways to use them that I recommend you go for.

Action Step

Get something which contains all of these particular Tonic Herbs. I highly recommend a Tea blend, but of course if that's inconvenient to you then get tablets which contain most, or preferably all of these herbs, and **take them every day**, that's the crucial thing. The advantage of brewing your own tea blend is that the effect is more powerful and immediate. The benefit of using tablets is that they're easier, more convenient, and more portable.

If for some very good reason you can't consume them every day, then please promise you'll take them five days out of seven minimum for the duration of this program.

Recommended Dosage

For brewing a tea, an ounce of dried herbs, which is around 30 grams, is a good daily amount, up to about 3 ounces or 90 grams a day once you're used to taking them.

For tablets containing extracts follow the manufacturer's recommendations, but 6x500mg extract tablets a day is good, building up to as much as 18x500mg, spread out throughout the day.

If that sounds like a lot of tablets, that's why I recommend a tea – it's an easier way to get a decent dose. The more you have the more effective they'll be, although taking them consistently is more important than taking them in large quantities, and ultimately more effective too.

Taking high doses consistently is the golden ticket to rapid results.

Caution

What is a Tonic Herb? Put simply, the distinction between a Tonic Herb and a Medicinal Herb is that Tonic Herbs can be taken as often, in as large a quantity and for as long as you like with no detrimental side effects! In this sense they are just like a food.

Medicinal Herbs on the other hand often have side-effects if taken too frequently in large enough doses, and care must be taken in their use. Even some foods like garlic would technically belong in the medicinal herb category, as studies have shown that long-term prolonged use of large amounts of garlic can unbalance the two hemispheres of the brain!

However, as with any foods there is occasionally someone who is 'intolerant' to a particular herb, in which case avoid the blend and reintroduce the individual herbs until you isolate the culprit.

If you do have any negative experiences taking the herbs initially, this is usually just your body getting used to them, as it needs time to get used to anything, no matter how beneficial. Just reduce the dosage and increase slowly, over the course of days and weeks, and you'll almost certainly find that any initial detrimental effects vanish.

STEP 2

GREENS

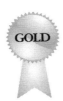

Description

Ideally the greens recommended here are going to be a part of your diet not just for the duration of the program, but forever. Greens have many, many health benefits, and there's nowhere near enough space to go into detail about all of them in this program.

You're just going to learn which ones you should have and you're encouraged to research and discover exactly why they're so beneficial, if you're interested. But, we won't go into it in detail here as it's not necessary. Everyone already knows that greens are good for you.

All you need to know for now is that greens are essential to curing your exhaustion, and in fact all healing.

So what are greens?

    1. Green foods

    2. Green drinks

    3. Green Superfoods

Caution

Now, you may possibly have some problems with consuming greens, especially with eating whole green leaves. A lot of people who have a weak digestion, and especially those who produce insufficient stomach acid, a common problem, are going to have problems digesting a lot of plant fibre, especially when they first start.

If that sounds like you then that's fine because, as outlined above, there are three different options for getting your greens. Ideally you would do all three but as long as you do at least one that's great – you're still on course to heal your exhaustion.

Green Foods

Description

When it comes to green foods, ideally you're going to want to include some green leafy vegetables.

Examples of green foods you would include are all the fresh herbs like fennel, parsley, tarragon, rosemary, oregano, sage, thyme and coriander, which each have their own additional specific health benefits.

Also all the standard greens you can find in any supermarket, greengrocers or market stall are great, such as: spinach, watercress, rocket, broccoli, cabbage, courgette, cucumber, celery, collard greens, mustard greens, arugula, chard, etc.

You should include as many and as much of these greens in your diet as you can every day.

Recommended Form

When selecting green foods the rules are:

The greener the better

If you look at some organic watercress and then you compare

that to an iceberg lettuce, one of them looks significantly greener than the other. You want greens that are really deep dark super green, not just mildly mediocre green. This means they are higher in an extremely important nutrient called chlorophyll, which you want as much of as possible, especially to cure exhaustion.

The fresher the better

As soon as a plant is picked or dug up, it starts to lose its life force, and it measurably loses nutritional value. This is why it's best to grow your own, or buy direct from the farmer. However don't worry about it too much: so long as it still looks healthy it's ok.

Always buy the freshest produce you can get. Shops will put their oldest stock in front of newer foods to get rid of it, but that doesn't oblige you to buy it. You can get the fresh stuff at the back. Eat it as soon as possible. This means going shopping more often, but it's well worth it.

It's the same with eating out. If you get served a wilted salad, send it back. It's rare that they won't have anything fresh, they're just trying to get rid of the old rubbish Don't accept it! As someone who used to work as a chef I'm very aware of this. It's called stock rotation: don't accept it. Also try to avoid any food which is reduced because of being old; it's rarely worth it

Organic is always better

With green foods, in fact with all foods, but it's particularly important with green leaves, you want to go for organic if possible. It doesn't cost a lot more in general and the amount of extra nutrients you get as a result of buying organic is definitely worth the extra cost however much it is, even if its two or three times the price.

Basically, if you've got £1 or $1 to spend on some spinach, spend it on organic spinach, even if you only get a small fraction of what you would have otherwise got for the non-organic version, because you're still going to get more nutrition as a result of doing that. Also you'll get fewer pesticides, fungicides, herbicides and other poisons that normally go along with non-organic produce.

Finally make sure you go for Certified Organic, or buy from someone you know you can trust. Otherwise 'Organic' is just a label that could mean anything.

Go Raw

Lastly, you want your greens to ideally be raw, meaning uncooked. A lot of the benefits of greens disappear, or at least diminish, when you cook them. With grains like rice, of course, you need to cook them and there's not a lot of difference nutritionally between cooked and uncooked rice.

When you cook greens however, you go from a food which is super nutritious in its raw state, to a food that's lost almost all of its nutrition as a result of the cooking process.

Ultimately, try to always eat your greens raw when you can. The easiest form of this: the salad.

Action Step

Am I asking you to just eat a bowl of salad? No!

The rule for implementing this is very simple: **eat whatever you want to eat anyway and just eat some fresh raw greens along with it.**

For instance, if you were to go into a restaurant and you decided to order a steak and new potatoes, have a big side serving of rocket and watercress with lemon and olive oil dressing, for example.

Or if you're at home, let's say you're making yourself some pizza and chips. Just make sure you have a big pile of greens, a pile of salad lettuce at least the size of whatever meal you're having, with your meal.

Always have greens in the house. Always order them to go with every meal. They need to become a staple food. What foods do you make sure you never run out of? Well, now include greens on that list too.

Recommended Dosage

The simple rule is: take your plate that you plan to fill up. On half the plate, put whatever you want to have: a steak, salmon fillet, pizza, pasta – whatever you're having.

On the other half of the plate put green leaves, like spinach, watercress and rocket for example. Now enjoy. Try to get into the habit of eating the greens first, or at least finishing them first.

Using this approach will give you a lot of different benefits.

One of them is that you'll digest the food you're eating a lot better, because it will have some fibre with it. Another benefit is that you'll have some real nutrition with your meal, which will help you absorb and assimilate the nutrients in what could otherwise be an empty calorie meal. A final benefit is that it's going to help alkalise you, and increasing your alkalinity will support your recovery from exhaustion.

Caution

There's a possibility you might not be able to consume whole greens. There are a lot of people whose digestive systems have become weak through decades of chronic misuse, and who therefore can no longer digest whole greens like salad, at least not without some discomfort or unpleasant symptoms like flatulence. The simple reason for this is that their digestive system just isn't up to it, although that will change as they get stronger.

There's a common notion that stomach acid, otherwise known as gastric acid, is just there to break down protein. This is certainly partially the case, but its main functions are to absorb minerals, to clean food and to break down fibre.

So the challenge, when you try to reintroduce high quality foods like greens, is that you may have becomes so nutritionally deficient, especially in minerals like iodine and zinc, which you'll learn more about soon, that stomach acid production is low.

These minerals and others are essential for creating sufficient stomach acid, and when you have insufficient stomach acid you may find that your ability to digest and assimilate highly fibrous food is lacking, because the levels of the stomach acid are lacking.

It's possible to supplement concentrated stomach acid, known as Betaine HCL, with every meal, which substantially alleviates this problem. The brand 'Now' do a good form.

Otherwise if this is an issue for you, don't worry. You can always fall back on option two to fulfil your need for greens..

Green Drinks

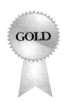

Description

Green drinks are an excellent way to get high quality hydration and nutrition inside you quickly and easily. They are universally beneficial, from people who have serious illnesses, to people looking to excel at sports, and everyone in between.

They help to increase the level of alkalinity in the body and neutralise acidic toxins. If you're exhausted you're very likely to be dehydrated, overly acidic and low in nutrition, and so you see how green drinks really are a godsend in every way.

Recommended Form

So what are green drinks? They can be either:

1. **Green Juices**

2. **Green Smoothies**

Green juices are simply fruits and/or vegetables with the fibre removed, turning them into a liquid, which makes them easier to digest and assimilate, especially for those with weak digestion.

Green smoothies are blended vegetables and fruits which

still contain the fibre, but it's blended down, which makes it significantly easier to digest and assimilate. They are also a handy way of including green superfoods in your diet. You'll learn about these in the next chapter.

Just to be clear: there's nothing wrong with fibre, especially soluble fibre, the sort found in vegetables. It's essential for health. But it's a strain on a weak digestion, especially if you're not used to having a lot of it.

Both types of green drinks can be handy as you can take them with you and consume them anywhere with a minimum fuss. Green smoothies especially can be an ideal, and very filling, meal replacement solution for those who want to eat healthily but are on the go all day.

Follow the recommendations in the Green Foods section when choosing your juice and smoothie ingredients: always go for fresh, organic, green and raw.

Action Step

You need to get yourself a juicer. It doesn't need to be a really expensive one: you can probably get one for $25 – 30 (£20 – 25). You don't have to spend a lot, although please do get a nice one if you can, especially if it will motivate you to use it. Include how easy it is to clean as a factor in your choice. Any juicer that you actually use is a great choice.

The next thing you need to do is start to juice cucumber and celery with it every day. Ideally, have this in the morning, after your morning water (see water chapter), and before breakfast. Immediately before breakfast is fine if you're pressed for time.

Cucumber and celery really is a magic combination to juice. Other people get more exotic; they throw in lemon juice, spinach and kale and all sorts of other green foods, but then you run the risk of finding it disgusting and undrinkable. You'd be surprised at just how delicious pure celery and cucumber juice is, with nothing else added. You can always add some apples to make it a little sweeter if you prefer.

Just cucumber and celery juice is actually really powerful. Cucumber is one of the number one foods for the kidneys and celery is one of the number one foods for the adrenals, both of the organs and glands which we're looking to build up in the case of exhaustion. If you do want to add something a little more hardcore, I suggest some fresh parsley, another excellent tonic for the adrenals.

You need to consume this in the recommended quantities every day without fail. You'll very likely feel the benefits of doing this immediately.

Also consider adding a green smoothie into your diet daily, especially as a healthy snack to take with you if you're out all day. These can be savoury or sweet. See the Information Resources section at the back for a link to an instructional video on making green smoothies.

Recommended Dosage

Green juices are something you should consume daily even if you are also eating salads at every meal. Make it a daily habit.

Ideally in the morning before you eat anything (just before is fine) drink ideally at least a litre (2 pints) of green juice.

This will consist of 1-2 cucumbers and 1-2 celery, depending on size. If you're really dedicated, drink two litres (4 pints) or more. Don't be afraid of having too much: your body will let you know.

If you find that's not doable for you, then at the very least drink a pint of green juice. Ideally, though, you want a litre. If you really want that massive improvement which we've talked about then you're going to be drinking a litre of green juice a day, for at least 90 days.

Also, if you're feeling especially stressed, tense or frustrated at any time, a green juice like this can have an amazingly calming and relaxing effect on the mind, body and emotions. It can also be used with children who are throwing a tantrum to calm them down, if you can get them to drink it!

See the Information Resources section for a link to an instructional video on making green juices.

Extra Credit

Two more honourable mentions in the green drinks category:

Wheatgrass juice

Barley grass juice

This recommendation is only for those who are of a particularly heroic mindset, so if it doesn't appeal to you then don't worry, you can skip forward to the next section.

Wheatgrass and barley grass juice however, which you can get from most of the smoothie emporiums which are ubiquitous these days if you live in a city, come in little espresso sized shots of juice.

They're like a super concentrated shot of liquid energy which can do wonders for your energy levels, both at an immediate level and on a long-term basis. They're also fantastic at cleaning you out, which is where the caution arises...

Caution

If you're dealing with a particularly high toxic load in your body, or your digestive system is particularly compromised, then there's a possibility that wheatgrass or barley grass juice may start off a 'cleansing' reaction in you.

This might mean you feel a bit under the weather or you may be excreting a lot more than you would normally expect that day. This is all for the good but it's not an essential part of this program, and it's up to you whether you want to ride out the cleansing reaction, decrease the amounts of the substance bringing it on, or stop totally.

The essential point of this part of the program is to have some green juice every day as described, and ideally a green superfood smoothie too. Everyone can absorb a green juice, at least the incredibly gentle combination of cucumber and celery recommended here.

Green Superfoods

Description

Green superfoods often come in the form of green powders, although you sometimes find them in the form of crystallised flakes, tablets, tablets, inside other foods or in a liquid form.

What is a superfood?

Simply, a superfood is a food that is extremely nutrient dense, meaning that ounce per ounce it contains far more nutrients than most standard foods. The opposite of this would be empty calorie foods like junk food, which contain little or no real nutrition, and in fact rob the body of nutrients just to digest them. So superfoods leave a surplus of nutrients, rather than robbing the body of nutrients.

The other thing which distinguishes superfoods from standard foods is that they have been shown to have extensive benefits to human health as well as standard nutritional factors, so that they could also be classified as a herb. Goji berries are an example that fits into both categories: it's both a tonic herb and a food, hence a superfood.

Recommended Forms

Some of the best green superfoods include:

Kelp: an incredibly high mineral seaweed usually bought as a powder. More info in the **Iodine** Chapter, coming up. Starwest Botanicals do an excellent Kelp.

Barley Grass Powder: a very nutritious and alkalising green powder. Starwest Botanicals do a great quality and very affordable version.

Chlorella: an algae famous for its high chlorophyll content and liver tonic properties. Sun Chlorella is an excellent brand, as is Jarrow's Yaeyama Chlorella.

Spirulina: another highly nutritious algae, with a very cooling effect on the body. Healthforce Nutritionals do a high quality Spirulina. Quality varies significantly depending on your source.

AFA Blue Green Algae: a super algae with all the benefits of Spirulina, plus active ingredients which improve your mood. Crystal Manna and E3 live are excellent forms.

Marine Phytoplankton: see below

All of these are excellent and you would benefit from including all of them in your regular diet. There are many companies now doing blends of all of these and many more, conveniently combined. Vitamineral greens and Lion Heart Supergreens are great brands.

I highly encourage you to investigate and find out more about them, as volumes could be written about each of their benefits, and in many cases has been. See the Information Resources section to learn more.

However, for the purposes of this program, let's focus on the most concentrated, powerful and useful green superfood of them all:

Marine Phytoplankton

Description

Marine Phytoplankton is probably the most nutritionally concentrated and complete food source available on the planet right now, which is going to be incredibly useful in recharging depleted nutrient reserves, and you are going to have very depleted nutrient reserves in your body if you are exhausted. Amazingly, it's also one of the most abundant life forms on Earth.

Marine Phytoplankton contains pure energy

What's special about **Marine Phytoplankton** is that it contains something called ATP, which is basically pure energy. You may know that calories are a measurement of energy, but you may not know that in order to use them, your body has to go through a very long series of chemical processes. These finally turn calories into energy, which is known as ATP, which then becomes pure energy. This becomes the movement of you breathing or you moving or you speaking or anything else you do.

It's all fuelled by ATP: not calories, not food - at least not directly. In fact adequate hydration and oxygen are more important for producing ATP, which is why you can go longer without eating than you can go without breathing or drinking water.

ATP is the direct precursor to that literal energy, often referred to in Taoist medicine as Chi or Qi. It's where matter meets energy. Obviously any source of pure energy that you can take in is excellent news if you're exhausted.

This is because it doesn't require the strain and exhausting process of extracting that energy from food via digestion, which is one of the top three largest energy expenditures that your body makes. That's right: digestion actually uses up a lot of precious energy.

You may be thinking 'big deal, if I need some extra energy I'll just have a coffee or Red Bull' or some similar stimulant. However there's a huge difference:

A stimulant uses up energy from your already depleted reserves. Marine Phytoplankton contains pure energy, so it increases your energy, rather than robbing your reserves.

Stimulants take energy away. Marine Phytoplankton gives it to you. Big difference, right?

That's the main reason why you want to be having marine phytoplankton every day throughout this program. It's not as essential as the green juice, so if you can't possibly afford it (it's reasonably expensive) you can get away with not having it.

Action Step

Buy at least one type of green superfood, preferably marine phytoplankton, and a green superfood blend, and take it in the recommended quantities every day. There are many different formulas out there which contain a ready mixed blend of some of the best ones. Any of the blends sold by the retailers recommended in the **Resources** section will be top quality.

Ideally you would get a green superfood blend, some AFA Blue Green Algae, and some Oceans Alive Marine Phytoplankton and have them in the recommended amounts every day.

Recommended Dosage

With individual green superfoods like spirulina, chlorella or green barley grass, or green superfood blends, you want to start with half a teaspoon a day (around 2,500mg or 2.5g), quickly building up to, ideally, a tablespoon or two a day, which is 10,000-20,000mg or 10-20 grams.

If you prefer taking them in tablet form because you find the taste objectionable, this is an option, but then you're looking at having a lot of tablets every day – anything between 20-40 tablets, depending on the size of them. This is also the more expensive option, but it's worth it to have an optimal amount if you don't like the taste of the powders.

In terms of dosage, the marine phytoplankton and AFA blue green algae vary a lot depending which form they come in. Start at the minimum **Recommended Dosage** with an eye towards getting to a more maximum recommended amount as soon as possible, so long as it doesn't make your body uncomfortable of course.

An Instant Boost

The marine phytoplankton is particularly handy in the liquid form which Oceans Alive does, as you can just put a few drops under your tongue and leave it to absorb for a minute whenever your energy levels feel low or your brain feels foggy.

This can often give you an instant boost. Try this before reaching for a coffee or other stimulants – you may be surprised! A client once compared it to a shot of espresso – without the energy crash afterwards of course.

Caution

All green superfoods, can bring on a 'cleansing' reaction, which is not dangerous, but can be mildly unpleasant. Basically, your body sees the extra nutrition as an opportunity to unburden you of some toxicity.

This is good news: you want it out. But sometimes it doesn't feel too good on its way out. Stimulants feel good because you feel the good energy as it's draining out of your body, and healthy foods sometimes feel bad as the bad stuff is leaving your body.

This is a simplified explanation but it's basically what's going on, and it can be very confusing unless you understand it. We're so wired to believe that what feels good, is good and vice versa. This is true, but only for a healthy body, not an exhausted one.

If this kind of cleansing reaction does happen to a degree which you find excessively inconvenient or uncomfortable, just stop taking the product until any symptoms stop and then start again on a lower dose – half as much as you were having before is normally good.

STEP 3

MINERALS

Description

Minerals are very important in nutrition, even more important to sustain life than calories. They are often overlooked in favour of protein, vitamins, antioxidants etc, but are actually far more essential.

Most of us are extremely depleted in minerals, because the plants we eat, and the plants eaten by the animals we eat, are severely depleted in trace minerals. Most food is cultivated with profit prioritised, so any mineral which is essential for health but does not cause a plant to grow bigger or quicker is ignored – which is almost all of them.

Research has proven that one of the easiest ways to predict an area's health is to look at the quality of the soil their food has come from.

Another factor is that some plants will take up and hence contain a lot more of certain minerals than others, even when they're grown side by side in the same soil.

Organic foods contain more minerals – from 50% to over 1000% more, which is an excellent reason to always get organic, but even a lot of organic foods are low in minerals. Wild foods are naturally high in minerals, and some easily available sources will be recommended here. A lot of superfoods are wild foods.

There are seven minerals which relate particularly to exhaustion.

Everybody's heard of some the vital minerals. Most people have heard of calcium and its importance to bone health (actually not true), and a lot of people have heard of iron and the danger of iron deficiency, anaemia (again, rarely caused by iron deficiency.)

Those minerals are certainly not unimportant, but we're not even going to look at them here. Instead we're going to focus on the seven minerals, usually overlooked or misunderstood, which are actually some of the most crucial for creating health and an abundance of energy because all exhausted people, and in fact the majority of the population, tend to be chronically deficient in them.

Most crucial in recharging energy are:

1. **Magnesium**
2. **Sodium**
3. **Potassium**
4. **Zinc**
5. **Manganese**
6. **Iodine**
7. **Selenium**

Bear in mind that once you are chronically depleted in a mineral, you need a therapeutic dose to get enough, and often foods are not enough to provide such a high dose.

Also, when you are very low in a mineral, your body sometimes excretes even more of it, or you may need a mineral to be able to absorb a mineral, so a catch-22 situation can develop. The end result is chronic and severe mineral depletion, and chronic and severe health problems.

This is why mineral supplements are often unavoidable, although a food form of each mineral is also recommended.

However, it's imperative that you get the correct form of mineral supplements, as most forms are worse than useless.

Caution

Supplementing minerals is a lot more challenging than supplementing vitamins or most other nutritional compounds. Most of the mineral supplements being sold are completely useless at best.

Most sorts of mineral supplements that we find in health food stores are in a form that's called colloidal.

This colloidal form is about a million times as big as the form which we find in plant foods, which is called angstrom sized. Plants get larger pieces of minerals and convert them into a useable form for us, angstrom sized.

The minerals you get from plants are also ionic, basically meaning that they have an electrical charge. This means that they're instantly useable by the body. Colloidal minerals don't have that charge, and even if your body can break them down it still has to give them this charge. Often it doesn't and just struggles to get the colloidal minerals out as quickly as possible.

If we could just eat colloidal minerals we wouldn't need plants, we could just eat our spoon to get the iron we need, or some pennies to get our copper. If only it were that simple. Yet that is what a lot of supplement manufacturers try to sell us.

A very common supplement, also used as a filler in all sorts of other supplements, is calcium, in the form of calcium carbonate or calcium phosphate. This is chalk, as in chalkboard. It's the equivalent of trying to get your iron needs met by eating your cutlery: ridiculous at best, and potentially very dangerous.

Recommended Form

So, if you're going to get mineral supplements, which are highly recommended as part of this program, make sure you get angstrom sized ionic liquid mineral supplements. They are in a size and form that your body will actually recognise as food, and be able to absorb into the cell to get the maximum benefit from the mineral without it clogging you up with large chunks of potentially dangerous amounts of minerals your body then has to struggle to remove.

These recommended supplements are water soluble and are always found in water form, never tablets or pills. You leave them under the tongue for a minute or so and they get absorbed straight into the bloodstream, avoiding the energy- consuming process of digestion altogether and benefiting your health immediately.

They are a wonderful addition to any health program, but you've probably never heard of them. This is mainly because the technology of making particles of minerals so small that they're the same size found in food has only recently become available.

The brand recommended for angstrom minerals is Mineralife. I like this one particularly as it has the golden triumvirate of: high quality, cheap cost and very effective dosages.

Before this form was available, chelated minerals were the best sources available: a colloidal mineral bound to an organic compound. That's a compromise which is vastly inferior to this latest innovation.

If you're buying standard colloidal minerals you're literally throwing your money away! Presumably part of the reason you've invested in this program is to know what really does work and what doesn't, so you don't waste another dollar or another pound or another euro on another useless 'health' product.

The only type of mineral supplements I recommend are angstrom sized liquid ionic mineral supplements, with the exception of MSM, raw salt and indium sulphate. There's an exception to every rule, right?

Minerals For Recharging Reserve Energy

The first five minerals listed here are primarily included due to their ability to massively build up the strength of the kidney organ system. This includes the kidneys, adrenal glands, reproductive organs and glands, the central nervous system including the brain and the bones, joints, tendons and ligaments.

They are also excellent for many other reasons. Previously I had also included another mineral, silica, but I found that it was less important than the others overall. The other difficulty was that it was really hard to test for it. To find out more about silica, see Extra Credit: Bonus Mineral at the end of this section on minerals.

Magnesium

Description

Magnesium is the most commonly deficient, overlooked and unappreciated mineral in the world. It's also the most crucial for us to have in order for us to experience abundant energy. Magnesium is involved in over 300 different enzymatic processes in the body.

Most importantly, magnesium is crucial in the process of manufacturing the all-important energy molecule described earlier, ATP. Without magnesium, production of ATP grinds almost to a halt, and you feel exhausted.

Common Deficiency Symptoms

include, but are not limited to:

- Anorexia
- Anxiety
- Asthma
- Brittle bones
- Calcification of the arteries
- Constipation

- Convulsions
- Depression
- Excessive urination
- **Fatigue**
- Growth failure
- **Low energy**
- Malignant calcification of soft tissue
- Menstrual migraines
- Muscular tension
- Muscular weakness
- Neuromuscular problems
- Stress
- Tremors
- Vertigo

All the problems that we've highlighted in terms of effects of being exhausted correlate very closely with the effects that have been noted as resulting from magnesium deficiency.

There is undoubtedly a very direct link between exhaustion and magnesium deficiency, and although it's not the only mineral you need, it is the most crucial.

HOW CAN I ACTUALLY TELL?

When you have adequate reserves of magnesium, fear and anxiety become almost impossible. You can test this with public speaking, unless this is something you're already accomplished at, in which case identify something you really fear.

If you feel no apprehension or nervousness before or during public speaking, then you probably don't need any magnesium. The vast majority of people will get very nervous at even the idea of speaking in public; many people are sick with fear. Most people are also seriously deficient in magnesium, and there's an extremely high chance that you are too.

Recommended Form

Magnesium is in a lot of green foods: anything that contains chlorophyll, which is the colour pigment in green foods, contains magnesium. As a general rule, the darker green the food, the better.

Nuts and seeds are also quite high, and the highest source known is a type of nut called cacao, commonly known as chocolate. However only the raw form is recommended, and not in large amounts as it contains a stimulant called theobromine, which you should ideally limit or avoid if you're exhausted, although it's preferable to most other stimulants.

All sea vegetables are an excellent source of dietary magnesium. Nori and dulse, commonly available, are good, but wakame, arame and hijike are excellent. With sea vegetables decent amounts do need to be consumed to experience real benefits: around 25-50g (1-2 oz) in a meal is a good amount.

Magnesium is also found in a lot of tonic herbs. These high-magnesium foods and drinks would form the basis of any optimum diet: greens, nuts and seeds and tonic herbs.

Supplements are the other recommended form, the best being angstrom magnesium and magnesium oil.

Angstrom minerals have already been described. In the case of magnesium they are good, but not enough on their own.

Magnesium oil is a special type of magnesium, Magnesium chloride, that comes in liquid form. It comes from ancient 150 million year old seabeds. You spray it straight onto your skin, and it is absorbed straight into your bloodstream that way.

It's excellent, extensively tested and immediately effective. Any brand that uses real Zechstein seabed mineral salts is effective, although again I particularly recommend Mineralife for quality and value for money. For more information, listen to the 'Miracle of Magnesium' interview which comes as a free bonus with this program.

Recommended Dosage

The more depleted you are in magnesium, the more of a problem you have with absorbing magnesium. It's one of those catch-22 situations, so the more you consume the better. If you consume it in the forms recommended here, you can't have too much as your body will simply excrete what it doesn't need.

The best way that we can get back onto the right cycle of having an abundance of magnesium, which relates to the abundance of energy, is to use magnesium oil.

There is **no upper limit** with magnesium oil: the more the better. This is an excellent way to build up your reserves of magnesium, which will definitely help you feel like you've recharged your energy.

The best place to spray it is on your calves, chest, hips, backs of knees, lower back, teeth, feet and under your arms. Make sure you spray an ample amount onto your skin twice a day.

As an added bonus you can spray it on any area of muscle tenseness or soreness for quick relief.

Action Step

Magnesium oil is amazing, so order it now. You won't regret it – you'll feel fantastic. Just this one step alone would bring a significant relief to your situation. In combination with everything else recommended to you in this program, the results you're going to feel will be absolutely incredible.

Cautions

With magnesium, we are generally so depleted that really there is no upper limit, at least not in the forms recommended in this program. Your body will just excrete whatever it doesn't need. In fact, the only caution is to use enough!

However, some people experience initial discomfort when they apply it; the skin may feel itchy or uncomfortable. Ironically, this is a great indication that you're really deficient, and that you need it all the more. But if it feels unpleasant, what do you do?

Start off by just applying it to the area below the knees, or if it's a very severe reaction initially just apply it to the foot, or just the soles of the feet. Keep applying it as often as you can throughout the day, until it no longer stings at all. Then you can apply it to other areas, and eventually all over.

Be careful initially, especially if you're sensitive, to not apply it to sensitive areas of the body where the skin is thin.

Some people occasionally experience a rash when first applying it. Again this is nothing to worry about. It's not an allergic reaction or a sign that something is wrong: it's just the magnesium doing its job and detoxifying your skin.

Remember that these occasional side effects are not a sign that something's wrong, only that you need more of it!

You may have tried magnesium before and not found it effective: this is either because you were using the wrong form, or because you just weren't using nearly enough.

Sodium

Description

Now this may be hard to swallow, what with everything you've probably been told about the evils of salt, but sodium is one of the most important minerals in the body, and you really need to focus on making sure you have enough, especially when you're exhausted.

Sodium is another mineral that your body uses up at a rapidly increased rate when your adrenal glands are overactive, or in other words, when you're stressed. What happens is the body excretes a large amount of sodium, and you need to replace the sodium in order to recharge your batteries.

The requirements that someone has for sodium when they live a relaxed lifestyle will be significantly lower than someone who has a stressful lifestyle.

So have you been lied to when you've been told that salt leads to high blood pressure and all sorts of other health problems? As is usually the case, it's more of a half-truth.

The crucial distinction is this: salt which has been cooked and processed is toxic to the body: it's unnatural and the body doesn't know what to do with it. It does lead to all those health problems we're warned about.

But raw salt – unprocessed salt which we normally find as Himalayan pink rock salt or Atlantic Celtic sea salt – is actually really beneficial to the body in appropriate amounts.

COMMON DEFICIENCY SYMPTOMS:

- Abdominal bloating
- Allergies
- Anorexia
- Apathy
- Depression
- Dizziness
- **Fatigue**
- Inability to concentrate
- Low blood pressure
- Low stomach acid
- Memory impairment
- Muscle cramps and weakness
- Nausea
- Poor protein digestion
- Stress
- Water retention
- Weak digestion
- Weakness

HOW CAN I ACTUALLY TELL?

Unfortunately, often you can't, and because deficiency of this electrolyte mineral is so serious, it's one of the first things that you're tested for when you go into hospital.

A craving for salt is an excellent sign that you have a deficiency or need for salt, but a lack of craving or even a dislike for salt should not be mistaken for you having enough. Have at least some salt every day, just to be sure.

A hair mineral analysis is more useful than a blood test, as the level in your blood will fluctuate fairly often, while the level your body excretes in your hair over months gives a consistent figure.

Recommended Form

The best food source of sodium is probably sea vegetables, including, but not limited to: kelp, dulse, nori, arame, bladderwrack, hijike and wakame. Celery is also an excellent source.

However the best source of sodium is Celtic sea salt or Himalayan pink rock salt, although the former is certainly better, and cheaper.

You can tell if your sea salt is the good stuff by whether it's damp and grey in colour. If it is, that's the one you want. Other types proclaiming to be sea salt you should avoid: they're still kiln dried and toxic, no better than table salt.

You can get these good types in pretty much any health food

store, as well as some supermarkets, and pink sea salts are pretty easy to spot as they are naturally pink.

You want to be consuming raw salt, so ideally don't use salt for cooking, roasting or any other heating process.

Ideally use salt in salads. You can have it in smoothies and you can put it in green juice.

If you don't really eat those sort of foods regularly (despite the advice of this program), then simply add it to whatever you're going to have once it's cooked and served. So if you're eating soup, stir it in the bowl; if you're eating curry or pizza, sprinkle some on after cooking.

This method is definitely superior to involving salt in the cooking process. This way you'll still get all the flavour of salt, and you'll also be getting the kind of salt which is going to be really replenishing and recharging your batteries.

Incidentally, a craving for salty food is an excellent indicator that your adrenal glands are depleted, and hence that your Adaptive energy is low.

Recommended Dosage

Make sure you have around a level teaspoon a day of good quality raw salt – more if your body demands it.

However, as you become less stressed and exhausted, your body's need for sodium may well go down, and less than half a teaspoon a day may be sufficient.

The need for sodium also varies depending on how much you sweat and how much you drink. The more you sweat and drink, for instance during strenuous exercise, which I don't recommend during this program, the more you will need.

Action Step

Take any cooked salt that you have in the house and throw it away. Do the same with any processed food that you have that contains salt in the list of ingredients, as you can bet anything it won't be the healthy kind.

Then go and get yourself some good quality salt, either the pink Himalayan salt or Celtic sea salt. Use it every day, as described.

Caution

Don't have cooked salt as it's damaging to the body. So no heat treated salt, and use the good stuff on your food only after the cooking process. If it doesn't make a point of stating that it's not heated on the packet, then it will be.

Cooked salt is cheaper to produce, so it will be cheaper to buy, but all salt is extremely cheap when you consider how little you'll use in a day, so this is definitely not an area where you want to be skimping at all.

Be aware that you can have too much salt, even good salt. Generally a teaspoon a day is a good upper limit even of good salt. If your blood pressure goes up, or if it's already high, that's a great indicator that it's time to reduce your salt, and/or increase your potassium.

Your body works very hard to keep the level of sodium and potassium in your body in the correct balance. Help it out by giving it enough of both in the right proportion.

As a general rule, if you've just come from eating a standard diet you have an excess of bad salt in your system, so you need to cut that right out and give your body a reasonable level of good salt.

If however you've been eating a healthy diet for a while, and perhaps even cut out most/all salt, you should think about increasing your sodium levels slowly.

Potassium

Description

Potassium, like sodium, is essential for the function of every cell in your body. Not having enough, or having too much, will kill you.

Generally, people are chronically deficient in potassium, and here's why: For the many hundreds of thousands of years we've been around, we ate mainly fruits and vegetables – precisely the foods which contain high levels of potassium. This has only changed relatively recently, just a few thousand years ago.

So we adapted to having a lot of potassium in our diet and our body excretes it very easily. Sodium, on the other hand, was generally scarce and highly prized, and so our body evolved to hoard it on a cellular basis.

Now most of our diets are exactly the reverse: high in refined salt and low in fruits in vegetables. Is it any wonder we tend to be low in this crucial mineral?

Heart disease, the most common killer in the western world at the moment, is directly linked to an excess of bad salt and a deficiency of potassium.

COMMON DEFICIENCY SYMPTOMS

include, but are not limited to:

- Abnormally dry skin
- Chills
- **Chronic Fatigue Syndrome**
- Constipation
- Depression
- Earaches
- Oedema
- Extreme cases, cardiac arrest
- **Fatigue**
- Glucose intolerance
- High cholesterol levels
- Impaired growth
- Insatiable thirst
- Insomnia
- Irregular heartbeat
- Irritability
- Low blood pressure
- Mental confusion
- Muscle cramps
- Muscle fatigue and weakness
- Nausea and vomiting
- Nervousness
- Poor circulation

- Periodic headaches
- Salt retention
- Water retention

Potassium is also crucial for clearing acidic wastes out of the body, and this is crucial because a build up of that acidity is one of the main factors that puts a strain on your kidneys, depleting your reserve energy.

Probably the easiest ways to tell are low or high blood pressure, water retention and excessive thirst.

As before, a hair mineral analysis is more useful than a blood test, since the level in your blood will fluctuate fairly often, while the level your body excretes in your hair over months gives a consistent figure.

Recommended Form

Generally, a genuinely healthy diet, as outlined in this program, can be sufficient to restore potassium to optimal levels. So much so, I didn't include it in the previous version of this program because I reasoned it was already covered with the emphasis on large quantities of green juices, green smoothies, green foods and superfoods.

Contrary to popular belief, bananas are not that high in potassium, but fruits in general are very high in potassium. Dates are particularly high.

Sea vegetables are particularly high, and they are also balanced with the correct ratio of sodium in general, making them perfect food for exhausted people.

Experience has shown me, however, that not everyone who does the program heeds the dietary recommendations. This is hardly surprising: the more acidic your body is, the more you crave acidic foods like meat, grains and processed foods and the less you tend to desire alkaline foods like greens and herbs.

So, if you're in any way not following the dietary protocol part of this program, it's advisable to include potassium supplementation.

You can get angstrom ionic potassium, and take it in the dosages recommended, or I particularly recommend a product called Rehydrate, which contains potassium, sodium and magnesium in a good balance. You just add that in the recommended amount to all the water you drink (see Spring Water) and you know you've got that angle covered.

Action Step

Follow all the dietary recommendations of this program, or get and use Rehydrate, or ideally, during the initial three months of this program, do both.

Recommended Dosage

Use the Rehydrate as recommended: around 1 teaspoon to a litre or quart of water is a good amount.

Follow the recommendation about green juice and sea vegetables outlined previously too: around 25-50g seaweed and 1-2 litres of green juice a day is optimal.

Caution

Be careful to follow the recommended amounts for supplemental potassium, and only use the angstrom ionic form. Other potassium supplements can be dangerous if used in vast quantities, and very large amounts of certain forms of potassium can even be lethal.

You can never get too much potassium in food however, which is why this is the best form.

Always aim to keep your potassium and sodium levels in balance. A hair mineral analysis will tell you how balanced these minerals tend to be inside you.

Zinc

Description

Zinc is one of the minerals we are most commonly chronically deficient in. Zinc is related to energy, fertility and in particular strength and power

The most powerful creatures on earth, in terms of how much they can carry in relation to their own weight, are ants. Some species of ant consist of something like 15% pure zinc, whereas a human being consist of only a very small proportion of zinc: less than 0.05%

So perhaps this gives you some idea of the importance of zinc. Basically the more you bring your Zinc to an optimum level, the more powerful you can be.

COMMON DEFICIENCY SYMPTOMS
include, but are not limited to:
- Behavioural and sleep disturbances
- Body odour
- Dandruff

- Delay in wound healing
- Diarrhoea
- Different kinds of skin lesions such as eczema, psoriasis and acne
- Growth retardation
- Hair loss
- Hang nails
- Hyperactivity
- Increased allergic sensitivity
- Inflammation of your nail cuticles
- Inflammatory bowel disease
- Loss of appetite
- Loss of senses of taste or smell
- Loss of sex drive
- Mild anaemia
- Post-natal depression
- Pre-menstrual syndrome
- Reduced fertility
- Skin dryness and rashes
- White spots on fingernails, transverse lines and poor nail growth

Most importantly from our perspective, a lack of zinc will lead to a sort of listlessness, a lack of willpower, which in Taoism is described as a lack of 'Yang Jing'. Again we can see that zinc deficiency very closely parallels with what we're told about exhaustion. In order to build up our abundant energy we need to build our zinc.

HOW CAN I ACTUALLY TELL?

There are numerous easy ways to see if you have a zinc deficiency. The simplest is to look at your nails. Are there any white spots? If so you almost certainly have a zinc deficiency.

An unpleasant body odour and a lack of sex drive, appetite or sense of taste are also good indicators, although they can relate to other factors too.

Recommended Form

Building up your zinc, once it becomes depleted, is relatively easier if you eat a carnivorous diet or an omnivorous diet as there's quite a lot of zinc available in animal foods in comparison to vegetarian foods. Despite this, most people are deficient in zinc whether they eat animal foods or not.

The very best source for zinc in animal foods is oysters. If you eat fish then eating a lot of oysters is highly recommended during this program.

If you're a vegan or a vegetarian and that's not an option for you, pumpkin seeds are the highest source of zinc in a vegan format. The only issue with these is that they really do only contain a small amount of zinc.

If you are someone who is highly dedicated to being a vegan or vegetarian, which is great, then supplementing zinc rather than just trying to get it from food is essential during this program to really boost your energy levels, and is a good practice for you to get into long term too.

Action Step

Get yourself an angstrom ionic zinc mineral supplement, Mineralife being the recommended brand. Alternatively, eat a lot of oysters regularly.

Recommended Dosage

A supplement containing the full RDA of around 15mg a day should be sufficient in most cases. But because zinc deficiency is so epidemic in this day and age, and especially among those who are exhausted, a dose of twice that amount, 30mg a day, would not be excessive for most people for the duration of this program.

Additional fine-tuning of dosage can be achieved by doing a hair mineral analysis.

If you are going for the oyster route you need to have at least 4 per day for the duration of the program.

Caution

Ensure your supplements are angstrom sized, not the colloidal form like zinc citrate, picolinate, oxide or sulphate (the latter is particularly harsh on the body).

Stick to the recommended dosages, and don't take more than 100mg a day of zinc.

Manganese

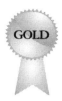

Description

Manganese is essential for energy production, and experience has shown me that all people with exhaustion and fatigue have chronically low levels of it.

What's fascinating to me about manganese is that the benefits of it sound exactly like the benefits of having an abundance of Reserve Energy, called Jing by the ancient Taoist:

- Better memory
- Stronger libido
- More energy
- Stronger connective tissue, bones and cartilage
- Better sex hormone production
- Fewer menstrual symptoms

We only need very small quantities of this mineral, but a little goes a very long way.

COMMON DEFICIENCY SYMPTOMS

Actual deficiency symptoms for manganese are so rare that it felt inappropriate to put them under this heading. They can be severe, but are unlikely to show up except in the most extreme instances. With the other minerals in this chapter, deficiency symptoms are fairly common and could be seen, from one perspective, to make up the majority of the severe illnesses that most people suffer from at one time or another.

So you won't really notice that you have a manganese deficiency, but you will notice the difference if you get it up to an optimal level: all the systems mentioned earlier, as well as your body's ability to extract energy from oxygen, fat and carbohydrate and your ability to use iron, will improve.

So while you don't feel manganese deficiency directly, you feel it indirectly, and it's an essential piece of the puzzle here that needs to be addressed just as much as any other nutrient, especially as it's so crucial for your body's ability to make energy.

Recommended Form

You find manganese in a lot of the foods that people most commonly eat, most notably sea vegetables, beans, fruits, greens and grains. That's why severe deficiency is rare.

However, the problem is often that the body struggles to assimilate and absorb all it needs. A lot is also lost through excretion, especially sweating. That's why giving it a therapeutic amount in a form that your body:

    1. Can instantly use

    2. Can easily excrete if it's had enough
                             ...is so important.

What is that form? You guessed it, liquid angstrom ionic mineral supplementation of manganese is highly recommended during the duration of this program.

Action Step

Get yourself an angstrom ionic mineral supplement and take it in the recommended dosages during the course of this program.

Recommended Dosage

In the correct form, a supplement containing the RDA, around 2mg a day, should be sufficient. Additional fine tuning of dosage can be achieved by doing a hair mineral analysis.

Caution

As before, ensure your supplements are angstrom sized ionic liquid minerals, not the colloidal form. Never take minerals in the form of tablets or tablets.

Stick to the recommended dosages, and don't take more than 10mg a day of manganese.

Minerals For The Thyroid

Whenever the adrenals are depleted and overworked, and they always are when you're exhausted, then the thyroid also tends to suffers equally.

The thyroid, among many other things, is the master regulator of the immune system. This is why when you get exhausted you also get ill a lot more easily. It's often because the thyroid is weakened, which sets off a whole chain reaction of other problems.

The thyroid is also essential for energy production in the body and regulating your body's basal metabolism. All the classic symptoms of low energy, low immunity and ill health tend to show up once the thyroid starts to function less than optimally.

Iodine

Description

Iodine is the most important mineral of all for the health of the thyroid gland. However, as always, it has to be the right kind: the wrong sort of iodine is highly toxic to the thyroid. Luckily, taking sufficient amounts of the right iodine will tend to push out the bad iodine.

The World Health Organisation considers iodine deficiency to be such a serious and prevalent problem that it assembled representatives from every country in the world to sign a document committing to ending it altogether.

COMMON DEFICIENCY SYMPTOMS:

- Breast, ovarian and skin cysts
- Cold intolerance
- Concentration difficulties
- Constipation
- Dementia
- Depression
- Dry skin
- Fatigue (most importantly)

- Frequent illnesses
- Glaucoma
- Goitre
- Hair loss
- Hyperthyroidism
- Hypothyroidism
- Inability to concentrate
- Infertility
- Irritability
- Low stomach acid
- Memory problems
- Menstrual problems
- Muscle cramps
- Nervousness
- Poor digestion
- Slow metabolism (difficulty losing weight and getting warm)
- Weight gain

HOW CAN I ACTUALLY TELL?

The easiest way to tell if you need more iodine is if you have trouble losing or gaining weight, if you are always cold, or if you get ill frequently. These symptoms normally go hand-in-hand with each other.

Recommended Form

Ideally you want to get iodine in food form and the best food form available is kelp. Other sea vegetables also contain high amounts, but research has shown they are not as well absorbed.

Kelp is a sea vegetable that you normally buy as a powder. Adding it to a green superfood smoothie is highly recommended, although you can add it to pretty much anything, even things you cook as the kelp won't be significantly affected by the cooking process. Kelp is the number one ingredient in Lion Heart Supergreens.

Kelp is also incredibly high in all sorts of other beneficial minerals and nutrients, including sodium and magnesium, and is very highly recommended.

If you don't want to use kelp in the quantities recommended, iodine angstrom mineral supplements are also great, although they don't contain all the other goodness that kelp does.

There are many excellent kelp powder products out there, although the quality does vary widely. Bad kelp smells quite fishy, while good Kelp smells kind of lemony. A great brand is Starwest Botanicals.

Always get organic wherever possible.

Action Step

Get yourself some kelp immediately, and start taking it every day. You can either get it in powder form or if you prefer you can get it in tablets.

Either way is fine but powder is preferable if you can stand the taste, because you'd need to be taking large quantities of tablets to meet the recommended dosage (see below), which can be a lot more expensive.

Recommended Dosage

Three or four tablespoons of Kelp in your diet a day, around 30g or one ounce, is ideal, going down to around 15g or half an ounce once your exhaustion is cured.

For iodine angstrom mineral supplements, follow the maximum recommended dose on the packaging.

Caution

There is no real limit to the amount of kelp you can have, so go for it. Your taste buds will tell you when you've had enough.

Be careful of any iodine supplements however. It's best if you avoid them completely, with the exception of the angstrom mineral supplements. Daily Multiple, recommended in the supplements section, contains a reasonable quantity of kelp.

Selenium

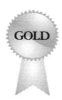

Description

Selenium is also included in this program to tonify the thyroid gland. It's the second most important mineral to take to heal this gland after iodine. It became particularly famous when it was discovered that people who ate foods rich in selenium were far less likely to suffer from cancer, and it's often supplemented as a cancer preventative nutrient.

COMMON DEFICIENCY SYMPTOMS:

- Age spots or liver spots
- ALS (Lou Gehrig's Disease)
- Alzheimer's Disease
- Anaemia
- Cataracts
- Cancer Risk
- Cystic fibrosis
- Fatigue
- Growth retardation

- Heart palpitations (irregular heart beat)
- High infant mortality
- Impaired immunity
- Infertility
- Liver cirrhosis
- Low birth weight
- Multiple Sclerosis
- Muscular Dystrophy
- Pancreatitis
- Pancreatic atrophy & fibrosis
- Parkinson's Disease
- Scoliosis
- Sterility in males
- Sudden Infant Death Syndrome (SIDS)
- Sickle Cell Anaemia

HOW CAN I ACTUALLY TELL?

It's not particularly easy to tell, but unless you eat a lot of wild foods and rarely get sick it's extremely likely you are deficient in selenium to some degree, as almost everyone is.

Recommended Form

The best source of selenium by far is Brazil nuts. Brazil nuts contain around a hundred times as much selenium as any other food. Brazil nuts are to selenium what ants are to zinc: they contain vast amounts so you don't need very many nuts to get all you need.

Another excellent reason to get Brazil nuts is that they come from a wild plant indigenous to the rainforests that has yet to be domesticated. So, every time you buy Brazil nuts, it's a vote to preserve the rainforest, through buying a food that only grows there.

Other than the special case of Brazil nuts, selenium can be quite tricky to find in food form, as it depends largely on where the plant is grown as to how high the selenium content will be.

Selenium is also available in angstrom ionic mineral form if you don't want to eat Brazil nuts for whatever reason. If your liver is weak you may be better off not eating any nuts at all.

Action Step

Get yourself some brazil nuts or a selenium angstrom mineral supplement. Consume every day without fail for the duration of the program.

Recommended Dosage

As part of this program you're going to have a few Brazil nuts every day: between 3 and 9 depending on your appetite.

Otherwise take the selenium angstrom mineral supplement, in the dosages recommended on the packaging, every day for the duration of this program.

400mcg a day is a good amount to have a day.

Caution

Selenium toxicity is pretty rare with this form of the mineral, although it does happen with the colloidal form. To be safe, stick to a maximum dosage of 600mcg a day.

It is definitely possible, however, to eat too many nuts. Try to limit yourself to a maximum of 100g or 4 ounces a day, and, if your liver is weak, less than that.

Extra Credit: Bonus Mineral Silica

Description

I've included this as a bonus mineral, not because it's unimportant, but because it's hard to measure your levels of it and see if supplementation is working, so I'll leave the choice of whether to work with it or not up to you.

Silica is pretty much unheard of. Out of all the major minerals crucial to health, whenever you look at a standard textbook on nutrition, you'll find mention of all the other minerals discussed in this program, and yet for some reason silica will always be left out.

Silica is in fact one of the most important minerals for you. It's one of the most important minerals for the kidneys, which are the key organs you need to strengthen to recharge your reserve energy.

Silica is one of the most abundant minerals on the planet, second only to oxygen. Ironically, it's also one of the least abundant minerals in our foods, because there are only a very few foods and herbs that contain silica at all in any significant quantity in a bio-available form.

Silica is also known as the primary beautifying herb, because it helps you to have elasticity in your skin and it gets your skin to be smooth and supple and your bones to be more elastic and not break so easily.

The common fallacy is that bones are built from calcium, but in reality bones are mainly built from silica and magnesium.

COMMON DEFICIENCY SYMPTOMS

- A sensation of heaviness
- Brittle bones
- Heart disease
- Lung disorders like emphysema
- Poor bone development and osteoporosis
- Premature wrinkles
- Sensitivity to cold
- Soft or brittle nails
- Thinning or loss of hair
- Tooth decay
- Weak tendons and ligaments

HOW CAN I ACTUALLY TELL?

The easiest ways to tell are probably the sensitivity to cold, a very common complaint among exhausted or stressed people, and the feeling of heaviness. When your silica reserves are high, you'll feel light as air!

The other symptom that's particularly obvious is tooth decay, a symptom that over 95% of people suffer from.

Generally, wild food is much higher in minerals in general and silica in particular than cultivated food – one of the main reasons why tooth decay and brittle bones are so prevalent in the modern age.

Recommended Form

The commonly available foods that contain the most silica are: cucumbers, radishes, okra, alfalfa, romaine lettuce, burdock root, peppers, tomatoes and oats. Of these, cucumber and radish are the most highly recommended.

There are a few herbs which are a much better source than any foods and these are: horsetail, nettle and oatstraw. These are the herbs that contain the highest levels of silica, and horsetail is by far the highest.

Horsetail is one of the ingredients in Lion Heart Herbs' Rejuvenate Herbal Tonic Tea Blend.

Silica is generally not available in angstrom form, but there is an excellent supplement called Orgono Living Silica, and that's another excellent way of supplementing silica.

Recommended Dosage

You need to make sure you are getting ample silica every day. You can ensure you are getting what you need by: eating the foods highest in silica, drinking herbal blends containing horsetail every day in the quantities recommended on the packaging, and/or taking the supplemental form in the amounts recommended on the packaging.

Caution

This is another mineral that you can't really have too much of: you will notice incredible differences in your energy, skin and suppleness through taking enough.

Avoid other silica supplements, unless they're an extract of pure herbs, as they tend to be in the un-useable colloidal form.

STEP 4

SUPPLEMENTS

Description

Although we would all ideally get all the nutrients we need from food, the fact is that once we are already depleted, we need all the help we can get.

The combination of growing crops on mineral-depleted soil, an excess of toxicity in our environment and a lack of freshness (many 'fresh' foods are picked prematurely, kept in storage for months and shipped all over the world) makes some kind of supplementation unavoidable as part of a optimal health lifestyle.

Caution

You must be very selective with the supplements you choose, however: over 97% of them are of poor quality, often containing nutrients which are not bio-available to the body at best, and they often contain toxic and undesirable substances like dicalcium phosphate.

Only go for the kinds of supplements specifically recommended, unless you're looking to become an expert in identifying exactly which supplements are actually safe to consume. Other supplements which would be very valuable but not an essential part of this program are recommended in the **Additional Supplement Recommendations** chapter at the back of this book.

Vitamin C

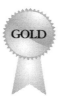

Description

Most people think that they're already getting enough vitamin C from fruit, orange juice or standard (Ascorbic Acid) supplements.

The challenge with vitamin C is that your requirement varies massively, depending on the amount of stress going on in your life and depending on how exhausted you are. The more depleted your kidneys and adrenals are, the more vitamin C you're going to be using up, and therefore the more you're going to need to get from your diet.

Vitamin C is one of the most thoroughly researched nutrients in the world. Doctor Linus Pauling, a famous double Nobel Prize winning scientist, did extensive research into vitamin C and proved just how effective it can be.

He showed how very high doses, far higher than usually recommended, can help some people recover from cases of terminal illnesses – terminal meaning that you wouldn't expect them to be able to recover at all from a conventional medical perspective.

Vitamin C is most famous for helping if you have a cold, and millions use it for that reason. It's highly effective for this.

Ironically though, it doesn't help you if you have a cold or flu by fighting off viruses and bacteria directly – it works by helping you to overcome stress.

Most people actually become ill because of an excess of stress, therefore they need much higher levels of vitamin C than normal. If you're stressed, exhausted or in a challenging situation, which everyone who reads this is going to be, you need, as well as the other nutrients we've discussed, very high amounts of vitamin C, which most of us don't get.

If you start to get these high amounts, your stress will go down to some degree, and you'll recover from your illness more quickly – sometimes immediately. This is how vitamin C helps to fight the common cold.

In fact, if you do become ill, a very simple way to get better very quickly, other than following the other steps in this program, is to take a tablet of high dosage vitamin C every hour. Especially if you're used to a cold lingering, you'll be amazed by how quickly you recover.

Unlike almost every other animal on Earth, we humans can't make our own vitamin C, so we have to consume it. Animals, when they are in a stressful situation, just produce more vitamin C. They can make it themselves out of glucose, a sugar that the body tends to have plenty of.

Vitamin C is especially good for the adrenal glands, so it will really help if your exhaustion is related to stress and anxiety, which it almost always is.

Recommended Form

Vitamin C is available in many different forms. Ascorbic acid is the most commonly available and the sort you'll find in any health food shop or any supermarket. There are other ones which are a little bit better, including magnesium ascorbate, which is a fairly good synthetic vitamin C, and calcium ascorbate, which is not as good.

However these are all synthetic forms of Vitamin C, missing all or most of the co-factors naturally found in plant foods which help it work properly. Ideally you don't want to touch any of the synthetic forms of vitamin C: what you want is a plant powder extract.

There are some plants that are naturally really, really high in vitamin C, so we can actually take those plants, extract them and get what is commonly known as 'food form' vitamin C.

This is a form that your body recognises as food and will absorb and assimilate easily. You often get less vitamin C in this form, but it's far more available to your body, and has been shown to stay in the blood for much longer.

The distinction is not quite as severe as the angstrom versus colloidal mineral debate, in that colloidal minerals are often not only useless but harmful. Synthetic vitamin C, however, is still actually quite effective, it's just not nearly as good as high vitamin C-containing plant powder extracts.

The top four plants that contain significant amounts of vitamin C in the doses that are going to help us if we're exhausted are:

1. Camu berries

2. Acerola cherry

3. Amla berry

4. Rosehips

All of these you can get in powder or tablet form. Healthforce do an excellent Acerola Cherry extract powder, as do Now, and E3 do a great camu berry tablet blend.

Action Step

Buy some supplemental Vitamin C of the type recommended, and take it every day during the course of this program.

Recommended Dosage

This depends on your level of stress so it will change as your life does.

Also, you need far more of the synthetic form than the plant extracts. If you take the synthetic form, ascorbic acid, it's good to start at around 1000mg a day increasing to up to 10,000mg a day and beyond.

There's a very simple way to tell if you've had too much of this form: you will start to have diarrhoea, or at least very frequent bowel movements. If this happens just reduce the dosage.

Interestingly this maximum amount will be considerably higher if you are ill, so while you may only tolerate 2,000-3,000mg when you are well, this may increase to 20,000 when you are ill.

With plant powder extracts take at least 1tbsp of the powder or 4 tablets a day, working up to 3tbsp of powder or 12 tablets.

Overall the advice is: take more rather than less. There's no toxicity no matter how much you have, and your body will get rid of any excess you have effectively.

Caution

The only side effect of too much vitamin C is that in really high quantities you may experience diarrhoea, although this only tends to happen with the synthetic forms, and is harmless, if a little disconcerting.

Daily Multiple

Description

There are many nutrients essential for health other than those already listed in this program. Every one of them is absolutely essential for the optimal functioning of the body, and they all work together in harmony.

If your body is healthy and high in energy, it can actually make quite a few of them itself. Specifically, research is showing more and more that if you have a healthy intestinal environment, with a majority of beneficial organisms (probiotics) living in there, they will work with your body synthesising what it needs to a large degree. This is probably why some people who are constitutionally strong, say athletes, can get away with eating a diet fairly low in nutrition.

However, if you're in a low energy state, then you certainly can't rely on this. You need to be looking at getting all those nutrients you need coming into the body. You can do that partially with diet, but as we've discussed, often that isn't enough.

You've already learnt about the specific nutrients you need to focus on to cure yourself of exhaustion, but what about your general needs?

In the first edition of this program I didn't include a multivitamin and mineral formula simply because I hadn't found one that was high quality enough to be worthwhile, or it was high quality but the doses were too insignificant relative to cost to be worthwhile, That's now changed.

Recommended Form

When choosing a multi formula, you want to look for something that contains all the nutrients you need. Obviously if you're exhausted, as explained previously, you're going to need more of specific nutrients.

Another thing you want to look for is that it's a whole food formula. This means that your body will actually recognise it as food, not a foreign substance to eliminate. If you try to put in all the different nutrients your body needs simultaneously, and they're all synthetic, your body just won't be able to handle it and will just eliminate it as fast as possible again, especially if it's already depleted and low in energy.

You want it to be liquid, not in pills and tablets. This makes it much easier for the body to digest and absorb.

It needs to taste good enough that you'll actually be willing to use it every day. Sure you may be a Spartan type who thrives on discomfort when you're in the mood to be healthy, but how long does that mood usually last? It's more advisable just to take it easy on yourself, and give yourself something you like wherever possible.

Lastly, you want it to be free of any unnatural toxic or harmful fillers, binders, preservatives, additives, colourings etc. This one is really important. Most people don't realise that the harm caused by the additives in their supplement pills often far outweighs the benefits of taking them.

The only multi supplement I've found that meets all these criteria is Daily Multiple by Mineralife, which is of course highly recommended. Any other multi formula that meets all these criteria would also be excellent.

Action Step

Get online or on the phone today and order some Daily Multiple or equivalent. Consume daily for the course of this program at least, and ideally forever, or until you have reach superhero levels of health – at which point you won't need it, but you'll see the complete pointlessness of not having it.

Recommended Dosage

Use in the dosage recommended on the packaging, but frankly you can have a lot more without it being of any detriment to you if you feel you need it. The recommendation is one teaspoon a day, but you can happily go up to ten times that amount with absolutely no toxicity or ill effect – another advantage of using a whole food supplement.

Caution

The only real cautions are the ones already listed: make sure the multivitamin and mineral formula you go for meets all the criteria listed earlier.

Also, be careful not to think that this will meet all your nutritional needs. People who are exhausted need way more of some nutrients, like the ones listed earlier, than they do of some others. So while this gives you a nice baseline to avoid any major deficiencies in almost all the main nutrients, it's never going to meet your needs for, say, magnesium, essential fats or calories.

Man cannot live on supplements alone.

Pregnenolone

Description

Pregnenolone is the root building block of all steroid hormones in our body, but don't be put off by the word steroids. Well-known steroid hormones include testosterone, DHEA, oestrogen and progesterone.

You've probably already heard how important it is to have a good balance, especially if you're a lady approaching the menopause. Whether you're a man or woman, it's vitally important to have a good balance of hormones.

What pregnenolone does is that it provides your body with the building blocks necessary to build all these steroid hormones. People often suffer from a depletion of these hormones, especially if their liver is not functioning optimally, or if they're vegetarian.

Men tend to suffer from a depletion of testosterone and women tend to suffer from a depletion of progesterone. An excess of oestrogen in either sex is also common and undesirable.

Normal hormonal levels often get especially depleted in people who don't eat meat. If you're a vegan or vegetarian you should be aware that one of the things which that sort of diet lacks is cholesterol, which your body makes these steroid hormones out of.

You can create your own cholesterol, but whether your body makes enough, and whether you utilise it properly, varies, and all these processes tend to be a struggle when you're exhausted.

Taking supplemental pregnenolone is basically cutting out the middle man, cutting out any need for dietary cholesterol and just giving your body the basic building blocks to make all those other hormones out of.

You can supplement with the actual hormones, DHEA being a popular example of this, but those kinds of supplements are risky – it's a bad idea to change a particular hormone level in your body unless you know exactly what you're doing.

Pregnenolone is safe as your body can make any hormones it needs out of it, and it can simply discard any it doesn't need.

Pregnenolone often reduces the craving for meats and dairy products, which is great as they often slow the speed of your recovery down due to them being hard to digest and high in concentrated quantities of all kinds of toxins and parasites.

Pregnenolone is well known for reducing stress, for increasing memory and for improving mood and energy levels. In fact, like magnesium, all its benefits reflect exactly the benefits of building up the strength of the kidney organ system.

Recommended Form

In supplement form, tablets are recommended. Source Naturals do a good product.

Pregnenolone is naturally extracted from coconut oil, and coconut oil is the best food source available.

Action Step

Buy some supplemental pregnenolone immediately and take it every day during the course of this program. Observe the beneficial effects.

Recommended Dosage

Take 25mg a day during the course of this program.

Caution

Always stick to the recommended daily dosage, usually one 25mg tablet a day. It is possible to have too much, although 25mg is a safe dose, and pregnenolone is a lot safer than other hormonal supplements like DHEA or testosterone, which can potentially have dangerous side effects.

STEP 5

HABITS

Description

Habits are the foundation that all of what makes up your life is built on. People think that dramatic events rule their destiny and determine what will happen to them. Occasionally this is true, but more often than not it's their habits that undo them, and it's their habits that lead them to success.

Think of it like a ship. Sure, the destiny of a ship is occasionally decided by a dramatic event like a storm or an iceberg. However the vast majority of the time the course of a ship is set by the subtle tides and undercurrents, the almost imperceptibly gentle breeze, and most importantly, *how we steer our ship in relation to these subtle but powerful forces.*

Consider this: How well are you steering your vessel –your body – in relation to what you want to achieve or experience in life? Do your habits support or hinder you in reaching your destination? Do your habits help you to go along with the flow of life, or does it feel as if you're always fighting against the tide, swimming upstream?

If at least the majority of your habits aren't supporting your journey, I have some bad news for you: you'll probably never reach your destination. And if you do you'll question if it was worth it, as you've had to struggle so hard the whole way. Of course, maybe you enjoy struggle, but let me share something important with you about relentless struggle: it's *exhausting!*

It's infinitely preferable and fulfilling to have your habits support your journey through life and lead you effortlessly to fulfilling your goals.

So how do you change your habits so they lead you effortlessly to your goals?

That question is answered in depth in my very popular bonus booklet **'Brand New Day, Brand New You.'**

If you do struggle to implement new habits into your life, it's highly recommended that you read this booklet immediately. It won't take long and the information in there is invaluable.

In this part of the course you're going to learn seven vitally important habits to support you in curing your exhaustion and experiencing abundant reserves of energy. Do them all, every day, and you won't believe the difference.

Caution

Don't punish yourself if you don't succeed in changing your habits straight away... especially if you're exhausted. Changing your habits requires the kind of energy which exhaustion depletes you of. For more information, and a strategy to get you started on the right track that really works no matter how depleted you are, see **Brand New Day, Brand New You.**

Grounding

Description

The latest cutting-edge scientific experiments have shown that it's really, really important for your bare skin to be actually touching either the earth or something that is earthed – that conducts the Earth's energy – for a minimum of 40 minutes a day, and ideally for as much of the day as possible.

So what does it mean to be grounded, to be earthed? If your skin touches dirt on the ground outside, if it touches a living organism like a tree or a plant, if you touch any natural water like a river or a lake or the sea, if you touch any mineral thing like stones or rocks and even if you touch concrete (although not asphalt, which they usually make roads out of) – straight away, you're going to be grounding yourself.

It turns out that, as Taoist have always known, one of the main problems for a modern 'civilised' human being is that we tend to spend most of our lives ungrounded.

We live in houses that are carpeted or otherwise insulated from the Earth, so we're not directly touching the earth. Even if we do go outside we tend to be wearing rubber-soled shoes, and that rubber sole stops us from ever actually connecting physically with the earth.

This is one of the main reasons why we feel so great when they go to the beach or the park, which so many people do at the first sign of a day off and good weather. We feel so great for many reasons when we do this, but one of the most important is simply: we're grounded.

One of the problems, from a scientific point of view, of not sleeping on the earth especially, and not having any contact with the earth generally, is that we build up an unhealthy electrical charge, something like static, and over time this charge decreases the functioning of our body.

From a Taoist point of view, and more and more also from a conventional western medical perspective, our body is basically a bioelectrical system. Our 'meridians,' a term commonly used in acupuncture and essential to understanding Taoist medicine, are like circuits.

In order to experience health, you want to actually ground all those circuits just like you want to ground any other piece of electrical equipment you might have. Otherwise there's a possibility that the charge can build up and eventually can cause the body or appliance to blow up, or at least malfunction or shut down.

This process, where the body's circuits overload, is commonly known as a stroke or aneurism, where the electrical activity just goes completely haywire in the central nervous system. This is one of the biggest killers of the modern age.

The heart is also basically a pump run by electricity. (Remember the paddles they use to revive someone whose heart has stopped beating?) Over 50% of people in the western world die of a stroke or cardiac incident.

Also, a lot of mental illness and all sorts of other problems can be traced to a lack of grounding. Of course, there are a lot of different issues that go into any problem as complex as the ones I just mentioned, and we rarely find one cause, but a series of factors which contribute to an event occurring.

These factors are like a recipe though: take away one ingredient, like being ungrounded, and you won't be able to make the dish.

When we are disconnected from the earth we build up something known as free radicals, which you've probably already heard of. In fact any of life's activities lead to a proliferation of free radicals in the body. This causes all sorts of problems, including inflammation and premature aging.

The question is: what do we do about them?

The way we're normally taught to deal with free radicals is to take antioxidants, substances which counteract and neutralise and eventually disarm these free radicals and stop them causing any more damage. These antioxidants are the colour pigments in foods. The more deeply coloured the foods the higher they'll be in antioxidants.

The best source of antioxidants, it's recently been discovered, was right under our noses all along. Planet Earth has an absolutely vast reservoir of 'free electrons' – particles with a negative charge – which conduct into our body as soon as we touch the Earth. They then instantly neutralise the free radicals.

The effect is instantly registered, although a deep level of healing can take several months depending on how long we've been cut off from our 'root'.

Recommended Form

Ideally your skin would be in contact with the Earth for the majority of the day and night. The reality is that this is almost certainly not going to happen, especially if you're a busy person living in an urban environment. It's just not practical. So what do you do?

The solution comes in the form of a grounding sheet, which is a very recently created and substantially researched piece of technology. You lay it on your bed, plug it into your wall, and then go to sleep on it.

This means that you can be getting healthier, reducing inflammation and replenishing your reserve energy straight from the Earth, all while you're sleeping in your normal comfortable bed. Does that sound good to you?

What a grounding sheet does is that it carries a charge from the earth up through a wire into your house and right into your bed. At the same time, it also discharges negative energy into the earth. So a grounding sheet is basically a sheet you sleep on, which is connected to the earth outside, and the result is that it's as if you were sleeping on the earth itself, although it's a lot more comfortable.

You may not notice the benefits immediately, unless you have chronic pain and/or insomnia, in which case you probably will. Its ability to relieve conditions like this is well documented and truly extraordinary.

It has been proven to help people with insomnia. If you have problems sleeping, where you keep waking up throughout the night, this is often because you're in pain due to inflammation. Extensive testing of grounding technology has shown that inflammation is radically reduced as a result of regularly sleeping on a ground sheet.

You can also get other grounding products, like a grounding mat which you can sit on when you're at your desk on the computer. You may have heard about the dangers of working with a lot of electrical machinery around you because again it will interfere with your body's bioelectrical circuitry. A grounding sheet will minimise a lot of the damage caused by electrical pollution – in fact it actually sucks it up in the same way a sponge absorbs water.

A company called Earth FX have done millions of dollars' worth of research on their grounding sheets, and that's the recommended brand.

Action Step

Get yourself a grounding sheet immediately. Plug it in, put it on your bed, and sleep on it every night.

Ignore your scepticism and trust me on this one. The price may seem high, but unlike foods or supplements this is a one-off purchase, and one of the most worthwhile ones that you can make.

Dosage

Preferably, sleep every night on your grounding sheet. This really is an essential part of this program, as odd as it may sound. Remember I said you were going to need to follow my advice on how you rest? Well, this is it.

It's one of the cornerstones of this whole easy exhaustion cure, and it is so easy because all you've got to do is sleep on a particular type of sheet. I can't imagine there's anyone reading this who can't manage to do that.

Alternatively, try to spend at least 40 minutes to an hour a day with your skin in contact with the earth. We have discovered through research that this is the minimum amount of time you need to be grounded a day to feel significant benefits, although if you're exhausted, substantially more is appropriate.

Get yourself a grounding sheet and use it!

Caution

Make sure your grounding sheet is on every day, every time you go to sleep. It only works if it's plugged in, just like your TV.

There is a possibility you might actually feel more tired when you very first use the grounding sheet and that is simply because your body may give you signals that it's really loving it and that it wants more time with this miraculous sheet.

It's possible that to begin with, even after ten or twelve hours' sleep, you still won't want to leave the bed. If this happens, don't worry. Go with the impulse if you can, and either way realise: it's not that it's not working – it is! It's just that your body knows what's good for it and it may not be keen on moving away from it.

Spring Water

Description

You may find this next step equally challenging to take on board, although it's easy enough to implement.

You need to drink spring water exclusively throughout the course of this program. What does this mean? If you drink water, or drink or eat anything containing water, it must be spring water.

Why is this? Because tap water, and to a lesser degree well water, are extremely toxic to you. This may well be the most important thing you do for your health ever, and I encourage you to make it a lifelong habit.

The water you drink is absolutely crucial to your health. Consider this: you are 60-70% water. You can go for months without food but only days without water. Consider this too: you are probably better off eating nothing but McDonalds and drinking spring water than you are eating organic highly nutritious food and drinking tap water.

Sound like an exaggeration? I'm not asking that you believe me, but TRY IT: try it for the duration of this program at least, and see how much better you feel.

You may have already tried drinking only bottled water and not felt any difference. But did you have adequate amounts? Most importantly, was it really spring water? A lot of bottled water is well water or filtered tap water —sometimes not even filtered. If you weren't aware of these distinctions, no wonder you didn't notice an improvement.

Spring water is magic; tap water is death. Those are the associations I want you to have.

After careful consideration I decided not to regale you with the horrors of the effects of chlorine, fluoride and nanobacteria found in our tap water, as I promised at the beginning that we wouldn't focus on the problem, only on the solution.

What if you have a filter? No filter is 100% effective. However if you have a really high quality one, that you've invested a lot of money in and that you trust, then by all means stick with that. But not during the course of this program! Spring water only please.

Recommended Form

What is the best form of spring water?

Ideally you would go to a spring and get your own water. That is definitely the number one choice, however if you're exhausted that's probably not going to happen. Perhaps, though you could enlist someone else to go and get it for you, say a week's worth at a time. Even if you had to pay them it would be more than worth it, and you'd be providing employment to someone!

Here's a list where there's a sliding scale, starting with what is the very best water that you can have and going down to the very worst sort of water you can have:

1. The very best water you can have is pure spring water from the spring.

2. Next, pure spring water in a glass bottle.

3. Next, pure spring water from a plastic bottle

4. Then filtered well water

5. Then filtered tap water of any type, and there are so many different types we won't even go into all of them here.

6. Lastly, the very worst water that you ideally should not touch, unless you really have no other choice, is tap water.

There's another factor that you want to consider when selecting water. You want it to have a low mineral content, because the minerals in water are generally of a colloidal form (read the description on minerals again if you need to remind yourself of what the problem with this is).

You also want your water to be as high as possible in hydrogen ions but this isn't something that's easy to ascertain. Generally, fresh spring water is higher. Check out findaspring.com to find a spring near you, and sometimes this site will even tell you about the quality of the water.

How do you select the best quality bottled water? First of all, it must actually state that it is spring water. This is obvious but most don't, because they aren't. Mineral water could mean anything.

Next you look at the back of your bottle at the **mineral analysis** section and check the total dry residue figure. You want this to be as low as possible, preferably lower than 100mg per liter. My current recommended brand is Isklar, which is Norwegian glacial spring water, and has a **dry residue** figure of 34mg. It's one of the most pure water sources in the world.

Action Step

Find yourself a supply of pure, preferably fresh, spring water that is low on mineral content. Make sure that you have a constant abundant supply of this water. Always be on the lookout for even better water sources.

Drink your water in the recommended quantities every day without fail.

Always start the day with a minimum of one litre or two pints of high quality water, before you drink or eat anything else. This is a must during this program. Adding fresh lemon juice and a pinch of salt to it will help it to be absorbed better. If you need to drink it warm to stop it making you too cold, go ahead.

Dosage

In order to truly cure yourself of exhaustion, you're going to have to be committed to doing something called **Superhydrating.**

Superhydrating basically means that you're going to flood your body with large amounts of high quality water and other liquids like green juices and Tonic Teas, as well as the correct electrolytes, until you actually start to hydrate your cells – not an easy job when you're chronically dehydrated.

Don't forget you will be chronically dehydrated if you're stressed or exhausted, no matter how much liquid you already drink. If you do already drink a lot then it probably just goes straight through you, or sits in your stomach, right?

Two litres of water a day is really the minimum you're going to want to have for the rest of your life. All the myths about too much water are just that, myths.

Realise also that the more dehydrated you are, the less your body wants to drink water as it actually shuts the part of your brain that asks for water down, and often you feel hungry instead when you should be feeling thirsty. All overweight people are dehydrated, and most underweight people are too.

The healthier your organs become, the more you can trust their signals (like drink or eat) but the less healthy you are the less you can trust them. *Just because you don't feel like drinking, doesn't mean you don't need to drink.*

If drinking that much water really is a chore to you, then it's all the more important to get your body used to drinking water. Get your body used to drinking at least 2litres of spring water a day, as well as all your other liquids. If you do hate to drink water bear in mind that that may well be because you're used to drinking tap water which is genuinely disgusting. Have a fresh start with spring water.

Caution

Tap water: Just say no!

Be aware of other things that tap water may be in. Always make your tea, coffee or herbal tea with spring water. Drink wine rather than beer as beer often contains tap water. What were the cows drinking that made your milk? What did they use to make the dough of the bread you're eating? Avoid tap water at every opportunity.

Some people worry about drinking too much water. It's possible to drink too much, but even ten litres (2.5 gallons) a day isn't a dangerous amount. The only problem with drinking an excess of water, which is way more than most people imagine, is that your electrolytes can run low.

Electrolytes are the minerals sodium, found in salt; potassium, found in fresh fruits and vegetables; calcium, found in green foods, nuts and seeds; and magnesium, also found in green foods and which you're supplementing. So long as you're following the program, over-hydration is not a real risk.

However, stick to a maximum of ten litres of fluids a day, just to be totally safe, and don't drink them all at once. Be sensible: push your limits, but cautiously and slowly. If you find it really difficult to follow these recommendations, build up to them over time. So long as you're heading in the right direction you're on track to reach your destination.

Sleeping At The Right Time

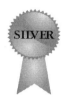

Description

Between 10pm and midnight your body does its main rest and rejuvenation of the internal organs, especially the liver, and the rest of the night not so much, so you want to be asleep during that particular time of night if possible.

Obviously it does vary a bit: it's not like some magic switch is flicked at 10 o'clock, but we're talking about around that time.

Certainly if its midsummer and it doesn't even get dark until 10pm then it would be ok to maybe go to bed a little bit later. However your body's circadian rhythms (your internal body clock) are aligned for you to go to sleep at around that time.

Before the invention of the electric light bulb around 100 years ago, most of us always went to bed at that time, for millions of years.

The important point to realise is this: often people who suffer from exhaustion never sleep at that time. How often are you asleep between 10pm and 12pm?

Recommended Form

The best way to sleep is on a hard, comfortable bed, with no electrical equipment on near you, in silence and complete darkness, in a well-ventilated and comfortably warm room, on a grounding sheet. This may not be possible but the nearer you can get to this ideal the more soundly you'll sleep, and the more rested you'll feel when you wake up.

Action Step

Sleep between 10pm and midnight whenever you can. If you still have things you have to do, you can always get up again after midnight and do them.

Sleep between these times as often as possible. Even if you work late and this isn't possible, you still have one or two days a week off, right? So try to sleep during these times on your days off.

Even if you only sleep between 10pm and midnight two days a week, you'll still feel a lot better. Anything is better than nothing.

Dosage

At least five days out of seven, if at all possible, make a point of going to bed at 9.30pm so your body can replenish and heal itself during these crucial hours.

Caution

There are absolutely no health risks associated with sleeping between 10pm and midnight.

It is possible to sleep too much, but where possible, indulge the urge to sleep a lot during this program. Don't see it as a bad sign if you feel like sleeping more. You're starting to relax, probably for the first time in many years. Take it easy on your body and allow it to truly rest. It probably hasn't done so for quite a while. Make it as easy as possible for your body to rest deeply.

Eating Early

Description

Try to eat your last meal of the day as early as possible, as this is another factor that can make a really big difference in overcoming your exhaustion quickly.

As a general rule, bear in mind that the earlier you eat, the more restful your sleep and the more likely it is that you'll wake up earlier feeling like you've got plenty of energy.

On the other hand, if you eat a really heavy meal really late at night, you can wake up after eight or even ten hours' sleep and still be exhausted. Yet if you go to bed on an empty stomach, so long as you're not so hungry you wake up in the middle of the night, you might get up after six or fewer hours' sleep, and just spring out of bed full of energy. Give it a try.

Recommended Form

Does this mean you must always go to bed hungry? No, but so many people think that something terrible will happen to them if they miss a meal, so even if they get home late and aren't really hungry they eat, because they think they should.

If this sounds like you then please just stop. Don't do it.

You'll feel a lot better the next morning if you just avoid the temptation and go to bed.

Action Step

Try to make your last meal of the day before 6pm at least 5 days out of 7. If this isn't possible, have it as early as you can, eat lightly, and don't feel like you have to eat to the point where you're stuffed.

Caution

If you have blood sugar problems like diabetes or hypoglycaemia, you may not be able to follow this advice. Work on keeping your blood sugar level stable as a definite priority, and perhaps investigate some long-term solutions that may be available once you've completed this program.

Breathing Clean, Fresh Air

Description

Fresh air is so vastly important. I'm convinced that one of the main reasons we get ill more frequently during wintertime is because we generally get much less fresh air.

It's so crucial for health to be breathing outside air as much as possible. In my experience, all other factors being equal, those who work or spend a lot of time outside always look significantly healthier than those who don't. Looking at the benefits listed earlier, it's easy to see why.

If 70% of your excretion happens through respiration, what do you think would be the effect of breathing the same stale air for hours or even days on end? Soon you, and your lungs, are literally drowning in your own waste, or the waste of others you share your space with. And, of course, all the goodness in the air, the oxygen and negative ions, are quickly depleted. This is why your mother always told you to go outside and play – it wasn't just because you were driving her crazy: she was showing she cared.

Recommended Form

Of course, not all outsides are created equal. Some areas have far better air quality than others. This is one of the reasons we always feel healthier in nature, or why beachfront properties are always highly desired. It's not really the view; most people don't have much time to be staring out of the window. It's the vitality: the oxygen and negative ions, that we really love.

So as well as being outside as much as possible, aim to make that outside as high in quality as possible.

The more plants, especially trees, and fresh natural water, like the sea or rivers, are in the area, the better.

The fewer cars, factories, houses – in fact anything man made – in the vicinity, the better.

Cold air tends to be fresher, and also higher-energy. The atmosphere after a thunderstorm, at the beach and near waterfalls is particularly high in negative ions and therefore desirable.

Action Step

Get outside for as many minutes of the day as you can, in as pure an environment as you can. Simple really.

If you're stuck indoors, always have the window(s) open as much as possible, for as long as possible.

But: what if neither outside nor a pure environment is an option? A reasonable alternative is to buy and use an air purifier and deioniser. This won't increase the oxygen, but it will at least clear away some of the waste and add negative ions back into the environment. It will definitely create a healthier living environment and, as a bonus, they tend to remove unpleasant smells: the main reason that people usually buy them.

Caution

There are absolutely no health risks whatsoever associated with breathing fresh air.

It is possible, however, to get too cold, depending on your climate, especially if your vitality is already low, so wrap up warm if need be.

Try not to let cold air hit naked perspiring skin, since this can easily lead to illness.

Relax

Description

This last point is probably the most annoying to you of all the solutions presented so far. I know that you're probably thinking, "Okay, not very helpful – if I could relax I wouldn't be in the state I'm in."

What's being advised is that you just be open to it happening! As long as you follow all the other suggestions outlined in this program, you may find yourself spontaneously wanting to relax, being more inclined to experience relaxing moments, or spend time doing relaxing activities – whatever that is for you.

If you don't know, maybe that's something you'll discover soon. For some people it's golf or fishing. For other people it's reading, or running, or yoga. Maybe it's just stopping at watching the clouds drift in the sky.

The point is, if you do start to get the urge to relax more, rather than feeling like this is a bad thing or like you're getting worse, just let yourself do it whenever you can. Go with it.

From a Taoist point of view, every goal-oriented, active, decisive step you take builds up your reserve of yang energy, and every bit of what I like to call purposeless activity, which is defined more by the attitude you take to it rather than what you do, builds yin energy.

Every bit of purposeless activity builds up your yin energy, and yin energy is always the type of energy that is severely depleted if you're exhausted, although both tend to be low.

You may be lacking yang as well – you may be lacking get up and go – but the reason why you're exhausted is because of the lack of yin. You may feel it as the lack of action and a lack of energy; you'll feel it as the lack of movement and all the yang qualities; but what's actually going on is that you've got a lack of yin. You've forgotten how to relax, recharge, rest and recuperate on a deep level, which is what yin energy does for you.

During the program you may end up spending your day doing very little: you might have all sorts of plans of doing stuff and spend a lot of time during the day watching TV, flicking through your emails and generally not getting a lot done because purposeless activity is actually what you need.

The problem is that when you fight against it, it tends to get even worse and you find it even harder to focus and get things done. Better to spend this unavoidable time doing things that are more meaningful than watching infomercials, like reconnecting with the world around you.

Yang is doing and yin is being.

One way of looking at this issue is this: Rather than always thinking about what you need to be doing (even treating sleep as a doing, because its recharging in order to carry on), just being yourself, just being with the world, just being with your environment, is actually really, really beneficial and really helpful.

Recommended Form

In those moments when you're inclined to just daydream or just stare at the sea or the sky, or go for a walk for no reason in particular: just do it.

It's reassuring that you don't have to think about why you're doing these purposeless activities. After all, if you did, they wouldn't be purposeless! In doing them, you are in fact increasing your levels of a certain type of energy and that type of energy is the type you really, really need for your full and total recovery. This isn't something you can force, just something you can allow to happen.

Just go along with the wisdom of the body in this case and let yourself just **be**.

If you feel afraid that if you let yourself stop and relax you'll be losing momentum – that you might collapse and never get up again – then don't be afraid. In the long run you will be much more efficient and productive as a result of taking a bit of time to build your yin energy.

Action Step

Action would defeat the point of this step. Just be aware that this is something that may come up, make time for it, and promise yourself you won't resist it.

Caution

There is such a thing as too much relaxation – too much yin energy – but not for an exhausted person. Don't go too far the other way in your philosophy on life: there is definite value in activity, focus, goals and all those yang qualities you've probably idealised for so long.

When you really see the value of just being, it's easy to forget the value of doing. Strive for a balance.

Everything in moderation, including moderation.

The Next Level: Bonus Habit Breathing Exercises

Description

There is a key part to this whole process that is completely overlooked by almost everyone. Even though I've been aware of its importance for years, I underemphasised it because I was convinced that acting on this crucial piece of the puzzle was just too difficult for most people. But experience has taught me that:

1. People **always** feel better when they act on this missing piece.

2. Most people are willing to implement it if they're desperate enough to get healthy, no matter how much internal resistance they may have.

So, enough build up: what is this crucial missing part of restoring health?

Restoring proper breathing.

What are the benefits? There are three main benefits which

you experience immediately when you experience proper breathing.

Benefit 1: You flood the body with its primary and most overlooked nutrient: oxygen. This has two main benefits: more energy and fewer parasites.

You have more energy because oxygen is an essential constituent to make cellular energy: adenosine triphosphate, known as ATP. Most people, when they need more energy, either reach for:

> **A:** A carbohydrate snack. This unsustainable form of energy gives a blood sugar rush, but then a crash, and is a vicious cycle often leading to insulin resistance, hypoglycaemia and even diabetes.
>
> **B:** A stimulant. This does the same as a high carb snack: raising blood sugar and then letting it drop. It also drains the body's reserve adaptive energy.

Really, you would be much better advised to do a few energising breaths and drink some hydrating water. Most of the time this restores energy and the need for food mysteriously disappears.

Most opportunistic organisms, including candida, and even cancer, thrive in an anaerobic environment. When you oxygenate the body, you make it a less hospitable environment for these organisms.

Benefit 2: You can truly detoxify. Did you know that around 70% of your body's elimination occurs through the lungs? A further 20% is through the skin, 8% through urination and 2% by defecation.

Yet in western alternative healthcare, most of the emphasis is in detoxifying is on the liver and the large intestine. Why is this? While these organs certainly shouldn't be ignored, I'd contend that most detoxification, in the actual literal sense of it leaving the body, occurs through what Taoist medicine would call the lung organ system, incorporating the lungs, skin and large intestine. When these are kept clear and optimally functioning, detoxification is pretty easy. When they are blocked it can be often be pretty traumatic, or at best it just takes **ages...**

The general view is that your body's circulatory system has a pump (the heart), while your body's lymphatic system, which is like your body's sewage system, does not have a pump, and for that reason you need to actually move and exercise.

I would contend, though, that lymph does have a pump: the lungs. Research has shown that there is no better method for getting lymph moving than the Rejuvenating Breath you'll learn soon. It's far more effective than anything else. When you breathe naturally, your lymph doesn't get blocked.

Benefit 3: Alkalising, or, more correctly, restoring pH balance to the body, especially the blood.

I've become more and more convinced that the theory that excess acidity is the root of much disease is accurate, but that the approach that is currently generally used – green juices, alkaline water and various bicarbonates – is very short-sighted. While it can be fantastic short-term, especially in emergency situations, this approach of just adding alkalinity can be unhelpful and dependence-creating in the long term.

Why is that? Because it's just treating the symptom, not the cause. Sometimes the cause sorts itself out, but often it doesn't. Then a new dependence is created, but rather than sugar, pharmaceutical and recreational drugs, the dependence is now on green juices and alkaline supplements. It's an improvement, but still a dependence.

I've been in contact with people who've followed this high-alkaline approach for years, or even decades, who still feel out of balance if they go a little while without a green juice or alkaline water. Then they start to crave other alkaloids like coffee, tea or tobacco instead. We crave alkaloids, the active ingredients of almost all drugs, when we're overly acidic and we need to be alkalised. This, and blood sugar imbalance, is the root of all substance addiction from a biochemical point of view.

So what is the cause of excess acidity? The organ system in charge of getting acidity out of the body is primarily the lungs, and the organ system for keeping the pH balance of the blood is the kidneys. If you tonify (strengthen) these two with various approaches you're really getting somewhere, and the benefits happen quickly.

Given all these amazing benefits to breathing properly, why don't we do it? Is it something we have to learn?

Not quite, it's actually something we have to relearn.

We all start off breathing perfectly: evenly, from the belly, using our whole diaphragm. We started breathing from the belly as that was our original source of all nutrients: oxygen, water and food, through the umbilical cord.

Then we were born, and at some point we were traumatised. This may have been at birth or afterwards. It may have been dramatic or subtle. But the bottom line is always the same. The muscles around the diaphragm become tense as they hold this trauma. And we start breathing from our chest in a shallow uneven way. Because we're always in a state of oxygen depletion, we tend to unconsciously struggle to breathe in, and then let the breath fall out.

Even when attempting to take a deep breath, we tend to breathe in slowly and then let the breath just fall out, exhausted by the effort. The Rejuvenating Breath basically restores balance by reversing all of these tendencies.

Recommended Form

Rejuvenating Breath

1. Sit down comfortably on a chair with your feet flat on the ground and the weight on your sitting bones, not on your spine. Hold your back straight and tuck in your chin. Seek out a yoga or Chi Kung practitioner if you're not sure how to sit comfortably with your back straight. It's possible to do this breathing lying down, but not advisable as the energy can tend to get stuck in the chest.

2. Take a deep breath in through your nose, with your mouth closed. As you breathe in, your abdomen, the area around your navel, will expand and go out and down. The chest should move minimally. Your body should stay as relaxed as possible. Your belly will look like it's bulging out. Again, most yoga or Chi Kung practitioners would be able to advise you on how to breathe this way.

3. Hold this breath in your lungs for as long as is comfortable. Concentrate on the area behind the navel for extra points.

4. Let your breath go out through your nose, as slowly as possible. This point is really key. After holding your breath for a long time, the natural inclination may be to get it out as quickly as possible. You need to do the exact opposite: control the breath to go out as slowly as possible. As it does your abdomen will deflate. But don't breathe in just yet! Really squeeze out every last breath with your abdominal muscles, until it feels like you've reached your absolute limit. Your abdomen will be almost concave compared to before.

5. Just allow yourself to breathe in. Ideally don't make any conscious effort to do so, just let the body breathe in naturally, completely filling your lungs. The effect is as if while breathing out you've been slowly pressing down a spring, and then you just release the pressure and let the spring bounce back. This way the breath in is totally unforced and natural. You may have experienced a similar 'breath for dear life' after being under water for a long period.

6. Then hold your breath again as in part 3, release slowly as in part 4 and breathe in as in part five.

Start by working up to doing ten of these breaths in a row first thing in the morning before eating, then three times a day. As you become proficient you can do more. I like to do 30 as an excellent way to start the day, and more later as desired. Many advanced yogis do this type of breathing for many hours a day, so there is no upper limit, but build up slowly and gradually to doing more.

7. It can be helpful to count along with the breaths to make sure you're doing them effectively. A ratio of 1:4:4 is ideal. This would mean that, for example, if you breathe in for the count of 5, you hold for the count of 20, and breathe out for the count of 20. This is only an example: it's the ratio that's really important. You can build up to doing a longer count as you get more experienced at this type of breathing.

Where to practise

It's really important to practise with a window open, no matter how cold outside, even if it's only open a little bit for the few minutes you're practising.

Action Step

Practising the Rejuvenating Breath every morning, ideally before every meal, will naturally start to restore proper breathing. You'll notice that, even in those moments where you aren't trying, you're breathing calmly, from the belly.

Your energy will go up massively.

You'll be more clearheaded.

You'll be more grounded and unfazeable

You'll feel better about life.

In fact, every aspect of your life tends to get better when you persist with these recommendations, because with more energy, and less toxicity and acidity, you start to come into the flow of life more, and all your other challenges feel less overwhelming and more manageable.

Caution

As already mentioned, you need to build up slowly in terms of how much you do, especially if you lungs have been weakened in some way.

It's also good to be aware that persistent practice of this technique can lead to profound ecstatic states. Doesn't sound like much of a caution does it?

The important thing to be aware of is to keep grounded. If you feel incredibly light and buoyant, simply ground yourself as you learned to do earlier. Ideally, ground yourself while you do the practice.

You may also feel more relaxed then you were aware it was possible to feel. Yes, just like with magnesium, this practice will make you more relaxed and more energised at the same time.

Other sensations, like a feeling of pressure inside, are also quite common. Just be aware that there's nothing wrong – this is a sign that it's working and that your vitality is increasing.

A NEW APPROACH TO ENERGY:

Breathe, Drink, Magnesium, Then Eat

When you're low in energy, don't think of food straight away, or stimulants, or rest.

These are inferior habitual strategies, which have led you to your depleted state. Here's the new paradigm – the one that will rock your world and bring you abundant energy.

When you feel your energy start to dip or crash, think:

1. I need to breathe

> Do your breathing exercise.

2. I need to drink

> Drink your fresh spring water.

3. I need some magnesium

> Apply your magnesium.

4. I need to eat

> Only do this one if you're still hungry after doing the first three steps.

This formula absolutely guarantees abundant energy long term

    Breathe

    Drink

    Magnesium

    Eat

It's so simple.

Just repeat it to yourself until it's a habit.

PART TWO

Storing Energy

Description

In Part One of this program, we covered in detail all the steps you need to implement to recharge your energy, and now, as explained in the Introduction, you need to learn how to store it safely. This part of the course is fairly small and easy to implement compared to Part One, because there are only two steps you need to focus on.

Once you've started to recharge your energy, the last thing you want is for it to drain away again. But unfortunately, this is what generally tends to happen. This is why often when you actually do get a few days or weeks off work, where you get to relax, go on holiday and are actually able to get sufficient sleep, you often may not really feel much better at the end of it.

You often still feel drained because you haven't really been recovering, since the energy that you could have recharged during a break, or during any attempts you've made to improve your heath and your energy levels, just drains away again.

It can be immensely frustrating, and it can make you feel like giving up. Perhaps it's caused you to take on a hedonistic philosophy where you believe that life is short and painful and you need to take your pleasures while you can, before it's too late. Or, if your character is more conservative by nature, you may even have started to despair that you'll ever feel good again.

This is one of the features that makes this program unique – that we're dealing with not just getting more energy, but keeping it. So pay attention and heed the advice in the following pages. It will save you endless pain and struggle, both immediately and in the long run.

Two Simple Steps

1. Astringent Tonic Herb: Schizandra

The number one Taoist tonic herb for helping us to save our reserve energy is schizandra. There are other tonic herbs which do this job too, all of which belong to the astringent category, including dioscorea and cornus. However, schizandra does the job so well that it's the only one recommended

2. Essential Fats: Omega 3 and Omega 6

Essential fats come in two categories: omega 3 and omega 6. Both, as the name suggests, are essential to health, as the body cannot create them itself, yet most of us are chronically deficient in at least one of these essential fats. There are other fats beneficial to health but they're not categorised as essential, simply because the body can make them itself.

STEP 1

ASTRINGENT TONIC HERB

Schizandra

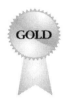

Description

Schizandra is possibly the greatest tonic herb of all time, and that is definitely saying something. It's the only herb in the world that builds all three treasures, tonifies all five organ systems and enters all 12 meridians. You don't need to know what that means; suffice it to say schizandra is a bit of a cure-all, and definitely one of the superstars of herbalism worldwide.

Schizandra has a huge number of benefits — far too many to list here — but one of the most important for our purposes here is its ability to conserve what is known as reserve or adaptive energy, traditionally called Jing. The depletion of Jing is the root cause of all exhaustion.

Recommended Form

Schizandra is the first ingredient in Lion Heart Herbs' Rejuvenate Taoist Tonic Herbal Tea blend and is available, in many different forms, throughout the world. It can be bought on its own too. Look for very strong tasting, sour, dark red, purple or black spherical berries.

Ideally you want to be taking schizandra in a tea form, or otherwise as an extract in tablets, whichever works better for you. They can also be eaten as they are, although the taste is fairly intense, and the process of hot water extraction (in other words, making a tea) helps to make the active ingredients more bio-available.

Mountain Rose Herbs do a good loose schizandra in the US and Lion Heart Herbs do a good quality whole schizandra if you're in Europe.

Action Step

Simply go now and get yourself some schizandra in either tablet or tea form and start taking it immediately, every day in the recommended amounts. There's no time like the present!

Dosage

It's always best to start slowly with herbs, so start with 2x 500mg tablets or 10g of dry herbs in a tea a day, and work your way up to a healthy dose. What is a healthy dose? As much as possible, within limits!

The main limit which is probably going to restrict you in terms of taking schizandra, is cost. If you're taking it as a concentrated extract in the form of tablets, you're going to be especially limited, because it's pretty expensive, but usually the more you have the better. If you get a bottle of 60 tablets, even if you were to have a bottle a day, you wouldn't be going wrong.

If you can only afford 2 tablets a day, that's also good. Ideally you'd want to follow the manufacturer's instructions. Most companies sell 500mg tablets, at a 10:1 ratio of extraction and you'll want about 6 of those tablets a day, which is the equivalent of about 30g a day of the raw herb.

Ideally you'll have at least 6x 500mg tablets a day, or you'll have about 30g (one ounce) a day of the Taoist Tonic Herbal Tea blends. If you're choosing not to take the other tonics, then you'll have 30g of just the schizandra.

If you're taking the Rejuvenate blend or something similar, then just 30-60g (one to two ounces) a day of the tea blend is enough. The other herbs support and enhance the Schizandra, meaning you don't need quite as much of it, but it should still be the main ingredient in your Taoist Tonic Herbal blend.

Caution

As with any herb, start slowly and proceed with the recommended dosages as soon as you've given your body a chance to get used to it. In the very unlikely event you really don't get on with schizandra, you can substitute dioscorea and/or cornus in the same quantities, available from the same sources.

STEP 2

ESSENTIAL FATS

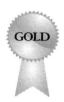

Description

The essential fats you need to be aware of are:

1. **Omega 3**

2. **Omega 6**

You've probably heard of omega 3, as fish oil. It may surprise you to know that omega 3, is generally something that is actually found predominantly in plant foods.

The only reason certain seafoods, generally oily fish, are high in it is because they eat a lot of algae, which contains omega 3.

This is the case, of course, with all animal foods. The only reason they ever have anything in them which is of any nutritional benefit to us is because they themselves are eating it, directly or indirectly, from a plant based source.

Caution

Getting good quality essential fats is actually quite tricky. Why is this?

Essential fats go bad, commonly known as rancid or oxidised, very easily and quickly. Or they are hydrogenated by manufacturers to keep this from happening.

Hydrogenated fats are even worse for you than rancid fats, although you can't tell they're bad by looking at them or smelling them. In fact, that's why they're hydrogenated – to massively extend their shelf life and keep them *appearing* fine.

So the first thing you need to consider, wherever you get your omega 3 and omega 6 from, is that you want it in a form which has not gone rancid or been oxidised.

How do you prevent this? First, you want to make sure that it's not already rancid by the time you buy it. It usually is.

Omega oils go bad very quickly when they're exposed to air (hence oxidised), sunlight or temperatures above around 100 degrees Fahrenheit. If they come with antioxidants inside, this helps to protect them to some degree.

Good quality omega 3- and 6-containing oils will be found fresh, stored in the fridge, in a dark container that keeps light out, and sealed. You would buy them this way then keep them this way.

They should also state very clearly on the label that the oil's been cold pressed and unheated. It's likely to seem expensive. That's because cheaper oils are cheaper to extract, and store, and keep longer. Unfortunately they are also poisonous to the body.

Hydrogenated or heated oils are everywhere, in almost everything, including most packaged foods, ready meals and restaurant foods. If you want to find it, simply look at the packaging and if it says any variation on the words 'fat' or 'oil' without making a big deal about it being cold pressed, this is a form of fat that is not nourishing, but poisonous!

For example: you've probably been told that sunflower oil is healthy. This is a typical half-truth. Sunflower oil, in its unadulterated form, is a great source of omega 6, but: the sort of sunflower oil that you get from the supermarket is completely useless.

It's worse than that. It's not just completely useless – in fact it's really toxic and damaging to the body. Why? Because it's been heated, and in the process of heating oils, especially oils containing omega fats (called *polyunsaturated* fats), you change their structure on a chemical, molecular level, and turn them from something which is nourishing to something which is poisoning you. It's an over-simplification, but it's a fact, and one that's becoming more and more widely recognised.

If you take an omega 3 or an omega 6 oil, and you heat it up to the point where the oil starts to degrade (above around 100 degrees Fahrenheit, although everyone has a different opinion on this – what's recommended here is the low end of the scale to be safe), then it's going to be actively bad for you, and from the point of view of overcoming exhaustion, consuming this degraded fat is another massive strain on your body.

Omega 3 Fats

Description

When we think of omega 3 we most commonly think of fish oils as the best source. The reason that a lot of people insist we need fish oils is because they contain a special sort of omega 3, called long-chain omega 3s, known as EPA and DHA.

There is some controversy as to whether you actually need this sort of long chain fish oil. Some people who are vegans say that actually you don't; you can get all you need from plant-based sources. Others say that you actually do need to get your long-chain omega 3s from an animal-based source.

The simple truth is that both are right to some degree: some people *are* able to make their own EPA and DHA, ready for the body to use. However, a lot of people, especially if they're depleted or exhausted, aren't able to do that anymore.

Anyone whose body is functioning optimally can do it, but for those whose bodies aren't, that conversion process often just isn't working anymore. They can't convert the medium-chain omega 3 fats found in plant food into the long-chain EPA and DHA that's usually found fish.

We **need** to have these essential fats in the right form, EPA and

DHA, in our diet: they are an absolutely crucial step in curing exhaustion.

They are crucial to the optimal functioning of a variety of things, including: memory; reducing inflammation; balancing PH; intelligence; mood; the central nervous system – they perform a huge number of functions.

But the most important thing they do from our perspective is to insulate and protect us: they store the body's energy at a cellular level. As previously discussed, we need water and electrolytes to conduct energy. Equally, we need essential fats to properly store energy.

Recommended Form

Flax seeds, chia seeds and hemp seeds, and especially their oils (as it can be hard for the body to extract the omega 3 from the whole seed) are excellent sources of omega 3, although not the instantly available long-chain version.

As explained earlier, the sorts of oils you want are cold pressed oils. You can include these in your salads or any other meals you're making which don't involve heating; for instance, you could add them to your smoothies. You can also add them to any warm meal, for instance a stir-fry or soup, so long as they're no longer too hot (hand hot is fine). Just pour some on the meal once it's served at the table, as you might do with ketchup or vinegar.

Remember this simple rule: if it doesn't say cold pressed on it, it's not. Cold pressed oils are harder to find, but you can still find them in any health food store and most supermarkets these days. Always get them as fresh as possible: if they are stored in the refrigerator when you buy them, this is an excellent sign. Udo's Oil is a very good quality brand.

If you don't already eat fish, then don't start eating it in order to get those long chain omega 3 fats mentioned earlier, because you'd also be inviting in a whole host of other poisons. This is well known now, especially about the bigger fish like tuna, which do contain omega 3. The governmental recommendation is to only have them once a month because they are so high in mercury, an extremely poisonous heavy metal, as well as a number of other poisonous substances like PCBs.

However, if you're happy to eat fish anyway, salmon, trout, sardines, pilchards, mackerel, and generally any oily fish are great. Something like smoked salmon is good as it's unheated; otherwise cook your fish minimally, although this is a tricky balancing act as you want to cook it enough to kill the parasites.

Fish often even advertises omega 3 on the packet these days when you buy it, and it's really easy to find out exactly how much is in it.

If you're vegan, or if you simply want the very best fish oils, and you don't want them to be rancid, then let's face it: often the fish you get in the supermarket isn't the freshest. Really you'll want to look at some of the superfoods and supplements as the best omega 3 sources. It's true that everywhere sells fish oil tablets these days, but these are almost universally rancid and contaminated, and are best avoided.

Marine Phytoplankton

One of the best sources of omega 3 is marine phytoplankton, for the simple reason that your body instantly absorbs it.

Because the EPA and DHA in marine phytoplankton comes along with substances called phospholipids, and because you absorb them in your mouth, the omega 3 goes straight into the bloodstream without your body needing to digest it.

That's really amazing news if your energy is depleted, as this usually means your digestion is not functioning optimally. To be able to get an instant boost of EPA and DHA straight into the bloodstream is great, especially when you have brain fog and need some help with memory, clarity and focus, among many other things.

Krill Oil

This is probably the best form of EPA and DHA of all, better because it contains significantly more than Marine Phytoplankton, but of an equally high quality.

Krill is a tiny form of shrimp. They are one leap up on the food chain from plankton, which are tiny single celled organisms. Krill are in fact so small, and they're so prevalent and abundant on the earth, that a lot of vegans consider it okay to eat them, as we're never going to run out of them. A substantial amount of the mass of all the life on this planet is made up of plankton and krill.

Krill oil is fantastic for building the strength and optimal functioning of the central nervous system, as is marine phytoplankton. It's highly recommended for anyone who doesn't have an ethical problem with it, and when it comes to overcoming exhaustion it's extremely helpful.

Both marine phytoplankton and krill oil come naturally with a very powerful antioxidant. Antioxidants are colour pigments that prevent free radical damage in the body. Krill oil comes naturally with astaxanthin, which is a very strong pink coloured antioxidant, and marine phytoplankton comes with a green antioxidant which is, of course, chlorophyll.

What these strong antioxidants do from our perspective here, is act as preservatives: they stop the oil from going rancid. Krill oil and marine phytoplankton are both also sourced from locations that are incredibly pure, so they're not going to be contaminated.

They're the highest quality of Omega 3 to be found in every way, and this is reflected in their price. They are worth it though, and it's far better to have 500mg of krill oil a day than 2000mg of rancid fish oil tablets. Quality over quantity is very important here.

Action Step

Buy yourself some cold pressed seed oils, like linseed oil, and use it every day.

Get yourself some marine phytoplankton and krill oil now, today, and use it immediately. Don't delay – it will benefit you immediately and it can take a long time to build up depleted reserves of this vital nutrient, so the sooner you start, the better.

Dosage

For cold pressed oils like flax or linseed oil (same thing):

Start with a tablespoon (15ml) a day, working up to about 4 tablespoons (60ml) a day, depending on your size. Don't forget that even though these oils contain a lot of calories they won't make you fat – that honour belongs to carbohydrates and cooked fats!

For krill oil: 2000mg a day is ideal. You can always have more – up to about 6000mg a day – but build up to this amount slowly. It normally comes in 500mg and 1000mg tablets, so that's 2-4 as a minimum amount of tablets a day, up to about 12 tablets a day. They are even better absorbed when eaten with virgin cold-pressed coconut oil.

For marine phytoplankton: with the liquid form, put quite a few drops under your tongue every day. Start with just a couple, and work your way up to 30 a day. With all these things, the more the better. The only thing that's really going to limit you is cost, because they're reasonably expensive, although not expensive in the grand scheme of things. You always want to start slowly and build up the amount you have over time.

Caution

Always start slowly with the recommended foods until you work up to the recommended dosages. Although you won't get fat eating cold-pressed oils, enough of any oil can be a strain on the liver, so restrict yourself to around 150ml of oil as an absolute maximum.

If you have any liver problems you may not be able to metabolise these oils at all, with the probable exception of marine phytoplankton. If in doubt or if you have any liver problems, always please remember to consult with a healthcare practitioner before proceeding.

After you are fully recovered you may feel less desire for omega 3 seed oils and more desire for omega 6 seed oils (see next chapter). This is a great sign, as ultimately you want to build up to a 1:3 ratio intake of omega 3 to omega 6 oils; that's one part omega 3 to three parts omega 6. However, during recovery you want to stick to a 1:1 ratio of Omega 3 to omega 6, as recommended here.

Omega 6 Fats

Description

Most people already have a lot of omega 6 fats in their diet from sources like corn oil, sunflower oil, soya oil and rape seed oil. These are the sort of oils that we eat a lot of anyway as they tend to be hydrogenated or heated to preserve them and then put in all our foods, often under the innocuous title of 'vegetable oil'. All our fried food is fried in this sort of oil. However, good quality omega 6 is still fairly rare in most people's diets, so it's still something you want to be aware of including.

Recommended Form

You can get these essential fats from eating hemp seeds, pumpkin seeds and sunflower seeds. These foods are really high in all sorts of other nutrients, including top quality protein, as well as the omega 6 fats. You can also get a cold-pressed version of their oils.

Raw seed butters, which are now commonly available, are a particularly easy to eat and easily digestible version of these seeds. They can be added to any cold meal, for instance spread on crackers or put in a smoothie.

Hemp seeds

Hemp seeds deserve to have the honourable mention. Hemp seed oil is the best source of omega 6 around, especially as it contains a type of omega 6 called GLA, which is particularly good for you. It's similar to its omega 3 equivalents, EPA and DHA, in that it's the long-chain version. GLA is the long-chain version of omega 6, which your body struggles to make itself and, again, may not be capable of making itself at all. So, consuming it in hemp seed oil saves your body a lot of work – always good when it's already low on energy.

Evening primrose oil is probably the most famous source of GLA, and a lot of the benefits attributed to evening primrose oil come from it containing GLA.

Action Step

Obtain some cold-pressed, fresh as possible hemp seed oil to put in smoothies, salads etc, or on top of your meal once it's served. Add pumpkin seeds, sunflower seeds and hemp seeds into your diet, perhaps as a cheap, convenient, delicious, nutritious and very filling snack.

Buy some today and use every day, forever, alternating between types every now and then to stop yourself getting bored.

Recommended Dosage

Start with a tablespoon (15ml) working up to a maximum of about 4 tablespoons of hemp seed oil a day and you're doing very well for omega 6's. Slightly less is fine if you're also eating lots of fresh seeds.

Caution

In order to preserve the omega 3s and 6s, anything that's been recommended that contains them needs to be stored away from light, heat and air.

They normally come in containers which filter out light, and they need to be kept away from air, so you need to make sure you put the cap or lid back on as soon as possible. They need to be stored ideally in the fridge, or at least a cool place.

These seeds and oils must be uncooked, not toasted, roasted, baked or anything else. You can buy seeds from retailers that specify that they're raw. Once you're used to them that way you'll soon taste the difference when they're not.

Ideally, all nuts and seeds should be kept in the fridge, because it prevents them from becoming rancid. You really want to aim to get them as fresh as possible. It's great to go somewhere which has a large turnover, and where you trust that the retailers are providing something of high quality. I recommend a few such retailers in the Product Resources section.

PART THREE

SPENDING ENERGY WISELY

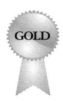

Description

From Taoist perspective, the reason why you are an ambitious person, a workaholic and/or an overachiever, is because you have a hot heart, or at least a tendency for the heart to overheat.

What having a hot heart basically means from a Western perspective is that you like to have your foot pushed down hard on the accelerator of life. It's not a bad thing, but it is an imbalance, and one that will mean that you have a tendency to 'burn out' more quickly than your colleagues who are more 'easy going' and less in a rush.

Just like with a car, if you constantly have your foot on the accelerator, the car is going to wear out a lot more quickly than it would otherwise. Now, does this mean you've lived a worse life somehow, just because you've reached the limit of your capacity sooner?

Maybe not. Maybe you've just chosen, by your nature, to live life 'in the fast lane', which is as valid a way to live as any other. It ultimately depends on your perspective. But as you're doing this program, it's probably because you've had your foot on the accelerator a bit too long, you've burned out your vehicle – your body – a little bit too quickly for your liking, and now you're wondering what to do about it.

That's what this whole process is all about: showing you a more sustainable way to live, not in terms of what you do, but by getting right to the root of why anyone does anything – the energetic situation of your body.

We've gone through how to recharge your energy, we've helped you to contain your energy, and now lastly we're going to take away the strong inclination that you may have, as soon as you're energy reserves get replenished, to just use it all up again immediately.

As a result of becoming exhausted, and realising you have no choice if you want to survive, you've probably put certain projects 'on the back burner'; you've probably cut some activities out of your life because, at the time, you decided they were non-essential.

Now though, as you start following the recommendations in this program, you will definitely, without a doubt, start to experience having a lot more energy soon enough. To continue the vehicle metaphor: you're filling up the fuel in your tank, and you've fixed the leak it had in it.

Then, the key question becomes: **are you willing to spend your energy at a more sensible rate?**

Answering 'yes' to this question is the key factor that's going to mean that you're actually going to have a cure to your exhaustion: a permanent solution. If you answer 'no', you'll probably need to keep coming back to this program again and again.

Please don't think you're being asked to resign yourself to a life of mediocrity or minimal effort. You can still do way more than most other people would dream of, if you wish. The important distinction is that you don't go **beyond your own capacity**, at least not as a matter of habit. If you do follow through on this program long-term you will soon find you have way more energy than you ever had before anyway.

So, to be totally clear, if you don't do anything else recommend to you in the program, if you only do what's been recommend so far, but ignore this Part 3, you will recharge your batteries and you will keep them charged for a while. But you will, almost inevitably, because you are a workaholic and/or an overachiever, push yourself too hard again, and ultimately end up feeling drained again.

But don't worry. We're going to solve this tendency once and for all with:

ONE SIMPLE STEP

Taoist Tonic Herbs For The Heart

Description

During this step, you're going to be taking a particular type of tonic herb known as Shen stabilising herbs. These herbs replace the lost yin energy in the heart, and this allows you to calm down and stop pushing yourself beyond your limit.

Now, if you're worried this is going to turn you into a boring or lazy, unambitious person, don't worry: it's never going to happen Being an overachiever is just the way you are. Using these herbs is just going to make sure you push yourself to your limit, not beyond your limit. So, you'll still have the tendency to excel and get to those peak experiences, but you just won't go over the top.

And don't forget, when you've got a lot more energy generally, you can actually expand your limits in a safe way that isn't detrimental to your health. But you have to go through a certain process to get there: every step of this program.

This is not to say you shouldn't ever push yourself beyond your limits. The problem occurs because most people who are workaholics and overachievers are pushing themselves beyond their limits day in and day out, and that's usually what's led to them becoming exhausted.

The herbs recommended for this step are:

1. Polygala
2. Albizzia bark
3. Albizzia flower
4. Ophiopogon
5. Asparagus root
6. Zizyphus
7. Biota seed
8. Poria
9. Reishi

All these herbs have so many benefits that it would take many books full to describe them all. You're encouraged to find out all about them and how they work if that interests you. See the Information Resources section at the back.

In combination, these herbs promote calm, relaxation, and most fundamentally a good feeling about life and yourself. When we feel better about ourselves, there's less of a desire to push ourselves to a breaking point.

This blend is also excellent at helping you gain a broader,

more expansive and inclusive perspective on life. This makes it easier to see what your own life is really all about, and what you need to do to start to actualise your full potential.

For this reason it's also excellent for those who are looking to end any addictive or compulsive tendencies they may have. When we see things in perspective, and we are aligned with a broader vision of the world and our place in it, then numbing agents like drugs, media and other obsessive behaviours like overeating lose their stranglehold over our lives. Although they may still have some place in them, they cease to be what our lives revolve around, as is sadly the case for so many.

This combination of herbs is also excellent for helping you get to sleep and helping you stay asleep. They do this not by knocking you out, but by calming the mind. Most people have problems sleeping either because they're in pain caused by inflammation, which the grounding sheet and greens will help with, or because their mind keeps racing and they can't get it to shut up!

Of course, if you actually believe you are your mind, then telling it to shut up so you can get some sleep might well seem impossible. This combination of herbs is really helpful for this. They help to still the mind, which means if you have something to do you can concentrate better, while if you have nothing to do you can relax or go to sleep.

The chatter of the mind, although entertaining, is rarely helpful. In fact, it tends to be exhausting! Anything which can get it to calm down, like these herbs, or meditation, is a real blessing.

Recommended Form

You can brew the whole herbs in water and prepare as a tea, drinking hot or cold, straight away or later on. The tea can be kept fresh in the fridge for a considerable period of time: up to a week. Lion Heart Herbs' Serenity Taoist Tonic Tea blend, which I personally formulated, is an excellent choice.

It's also possible to buy them and consume them in tablet form as an extract. Make sure they are an extract if you get them in tablets, otherwise they'll be a waste of time. You'd have to take dozens of tablets a day to get any useful effect, and many herbs have to be extracted in some way to be of benefit.

There are many other forms of these herbs, but these two forms are the most common ways to use them that I recommend you go for.

Action Step

Get something which contains all of these particular tonic herbs. I highly recommend a tea blend, but of course if that's inconvenient to you then get tablets containing most, or preferably all, of these herbs and **take them every day** – that's the crucial thing. The advantage of brewing your own tea blend is that the effect is more powerful and immediate. The benefit of using tablets is that they're easier, more convenient, and more portable.

If for some very good reason you can't consume them every day, then please promise you'll do five days out of seven minimum for the duration of this program.

Recommended Dosage

For brewing a tea, an ounce of dried herbs, which is around 30 grams, is a good daily amount, up to about 3 ounces or 90 grams a day once you're used to taking them.

For tablets containing extracts follow the manufacturer's recommendations, but 6x 500mg extract tablets a day, containing a 10:1 ratio is good, building up to as much as 18x 500mg spread out throughout the day.

If that sounds like a lot of tablets, that's why I recommend a tea: it's an easier way to get a decent dose. The more you have the more effective they'll be, although taking them consistently is more important than taking them in large quantities, and ultimately more effective too.

Taking high doses consistently is the golden ticket to rapid results.

Caution

What is a Tonic Herb? Put simply the distinction between a Tonic Herb and a Medicinal Herb is that Tonic Herbs can be taken as often, in as large a quantity and for as long as you like with no detrimental side effects! In this sense they are just like a food.

Medicinal Herbs on the other hand often have side-effects if taken too frequently in large enough doses and care must be taken in their use. Even some foods like garlic would technically belong in the medicinal herb category as studies have shown that long-term prolonged use of large amounts of garlic can unbalance the two hemispheres of the brain!

As with any foods there is occasionally someone who is 'intolerant' to a particular herb. If that's the case, avoid the blend and reintroduce the individual herbs until you isolate the culprit.

If you do have any negative experiences taking the herbs initially, this is usually just your body getting used to them as it needs time to get used to anything, no matter how beneficial. Just reduce the dosage and increase slowly, over the course of days and weeks. You'll almost certainly find that any initial detrimental effects vanish.

BONUS SECTION

IDEALLY DON'T

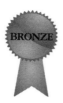

Description

You may be thinking: "Wow, a big list of things I shouldn't do – not much of a bonus."

I'll try and keep it as interesting and entertaining as possible, not the same old thing you've heard a million times before.

Now, you were promised we wouldn't be focusing on things you shouldn't do, and I've kept my promise, because this is it, I'm going to draw a line here. If you do everything that I've recommended above this line, and ignore everything below this line, you'll still get the results you were promised.

Ready? Here it is:

So don't panic. Just do everything that's been recommended so far and you'll do great. You will get better.

However, this program wouldn't feel complete if it didn't include a list of things that you ideally wouldn't do. These things that you ideally wouldn't do are not prohibited on any moral or ethical grounds: they are simply included because they're substances and activities that are in the category of throwing your energy away needlessly. The only evil, from the perspective of this program, is that which wastes energy, because that's what this program is all about – getting and keeping more energy.

Getting and keeping more energy is the only way to cure exhaustion.

Again, it has to be emphasised that you can succeed with the program without following these forthcoming steps. That's why this is the 'bonus' part of the program – the steps are optional.

It's also important to understand that if you do everything recommend so far, you will get healthier. Interestingly, the healthier you are, the more your instinct will be healthy – meaning reliable and accurate.

So you could look at it from the perspective that a lot of these recommendations are only there so that you have an idea of what is and what isn't actually healthy. Most people think they know, but a lot of people really don't. I had a client say to me once, in all seriousness, "I've only had a Snickers today, is that healthy?"

You're not being asked to try to force yourself to stop doing anything.

However, if as a result of following this program you have a natural inclination to do something unhealthy less often, then you mustn't think, "what's wrong?"; you should actually be equipped with the information to realise that you're doing what's right.

Of course, if you *have* been thinking of quitting any of these habits and addictions anyway, if you feel like you have the willpower and you're ready to do it, and if you feel like now would be a perfect time now that you've found out just how detrimental these things are to you, then by all means go for it. Quit and don't look back. But please don't feel that it's an essential part of the program.

There are six 'Deadly Sins' that you'll ideally remove from your life to cure your exhaustion, optimise your energy, look amazing, and feel great all the time.

They are:

THE SIX 'DEADLY SINS'

1. Stimulants

2. Sugar

3. Cooked fat

4. High protein diets

5. Processed foods

6. Sleep deprivation

If you conquer all these deadly enemies to abundant energy too, you'll feel better than you ever have in your whole life!

The Dilemma

It's an unfortunate fact that, at least initially, those things that drain us of energy make us feel good, while those things which drain us of poisons, thus allowing more energy to come in, often feel bad.

Why is this? It seems like it's simply because we actually feel what is draining out of us as it's draining out. So when we are drained of vital energy we feel good, and when we are drained of toxins we feel bad.

This is quite a thing to get our heads round. We may have learned in theory that sometimes we have to *delay gratification,* or go through something unpleasant to get a reward.

Despite this, however, we are obviously hard-wired to perceive the world in a certain way, and most of us do, most of the time. This hard-wired perception can be summed up as:

Good, pleasurable feeling = good

Bad, painful feeling = bad

The epitome of this perspective is summed up in the philosophy of hedonism.

The counterbalance of this perspective is summed up in philosophies like stoicism and martyrdom, where pain and discomfort are idealised.

Although some lip service is paid to these latter philosophies, most of us in the modern age are hedonists, even though we might not see ourselves that way. It's hard-wired after all.

Of course, self-denial is not what's being encouraged here either. What's being encouraged is that you become aware, you become smart, you make conscious choices, so you can live the best life possible.

Suffering for its own sake is a futile indulgence, mostly.

But delaying gratification – experiencing a little bit of discomfort so you can experience a lot of pleasure in the future, well, that's just common sense.

Stimulants

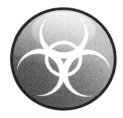

Description

Stimulants are one of the main ways that a person really drains their energy. The particular problem with this is that we are normally only attracted to stimulants if our energies are already a bit drained. Conversely, the higher your energy, the less you'll feel a need for a stimulant.

What is a stimulant? You may be surprised to know that a stimulant isn't just what you've probably been taught; it's not just speed and cocaine and other illegal drugs. A stimulant is any substance which stimulates the central nervous system, the cardiac system, and especially the adrenal glands.

How does a stimulant work? The answer to this question also answers the next obvious question: what's so bad about stimulants? The way a stimulant works is by being a poison. It goes into you and poisons the body, and the body reacts with alarm, because it's being poisoned! The adrenals kick in and they release neurotransmitters like adrenaline and cortisol, which increase your heart rate and your respiration; they cause blood to go to your muscles and your pupils to dilate; they cause sugar to be taken from your muscles and your liver in the form of glycogen and put into your bloodstream.

What's the upshot of this response of alarm? You feel great! Your fight or flight mechanism has been activated (because you've been poisoned) and you feel that much more alive than you felt before. You feel alert, awake and sharp, and you feel a sense of intensity. All 'peak experiences' even the psychologically healthy ones, rely on this fight or flight mechanism in combination with other physiological processes.

There's nothing wrong with having these peak experiences... occasionally.

They punctuate our lives and give our lives meaning; they can be very healing for our psyche, lifting us out of the mundanity of life. But, and this is a big but: **they drain our reserve energy.**

This is why most cultures have kept the situations and substances which bring on such intense experiences for occasional and meaningful use only. Do you see the problem with using this mechanism just to get through another day at the office?

If you can't get through a day without a coffee, tea or a cigarette, it's a sure sign that your energies are depleted. If you can't get through an hour or two without a stimulant, that's a definite sign you've hit exhaustion.

Common Forms

Stimulants include coffee, tea, green tea, chocolate and MSG. MSG is a really popular food additive which makes things which would otherwise not taste of much immediately taste really delicious. It's often labelled in food packaging simply as flavourings.

Alcohol is a stimulant: it depresses the central nervous system, but it's a cardiac stimulant, and it's an adrenal stimulant, so it's still a stimulant.

All the illegal drugs: cocaine, cannabis, speed, meth, meow, PCP.

Prescription drugs like Ritalin and its derivatives.

One of the most important is cigarettes because it's one that people have very frequently. Often when a person smokes, they are in a situation where they feel they need a stimulant more than once every hour.

For instance, if you smoke 20 a day, and if you're awake for 16 hours a day, that's at least one cigarette an hour.

As a result of following all the recommendations of this program, you will feel less inclination to have stimulants. Just remember that that's okay; in fact it's great. If you suddenly feel like, "Okay, I don't fancy my morning coffee" or "It's been an hour since I had my cigarette, but I don't feel like another one yet", don't feel like there's something wrong: just let it be, realise that it's okay.

Recommended Action

Identify all the stimulants in your life. Notice them: notice your desire for them, what prompts it, what alternatives satisfy it. Assess how you feel about being utterly dependant on these substances.

Most importantly, unflinchingly see them for what they are: poisons which give you a rush and make you feel good for a while as your body scrambles to get them out. Don't romanticise them. Don't kid yourself.

Whatever choice you come to about your stimulant use, accept it and become aware of the consequences of your choice without guilt or recrimination.

Caution

Often when a person tries to cut out all the stimulants in their lives, they will simply cut out the middle man and eat a lot of sugary and starchy foods instead. Although this is sometimes preferable, it's really substituting one drug for another, more socially acceptable drug.

Sugar

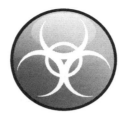

Description

Refined sugar is probably the most dangerous and addictive drug on this planet. Has that got your attention? I've had many friends and clients who gave up all other drugs – all the stimulants – with relative ease.

Sugar, however, most people feel that they just can't manage to quit. It is the real gateway drug, the one that leads to all the other drug addictions. I myself found sugar more difficult to quit than all the other stimulants put together. It made quitting smoking seem easy by comparison.

So what is sugar? Sugar is here defined as any unnatural form of carbohydrate. A list will be given in the next section. The problems with it are numerous. It causes our blood glucose levels to spike, which make us temporarily euphoric (the same as all stimulants do, remember?), and then our blood glucose levels crash, causing us to feel really bad. Some people become weak and faint, some turn into Mr Hyde, but everyone suffers – including the people around them.

What's the solution when this happens? Have more sugar. And so a vicious cycle of dependence and suffering continues that most people never escape during the course of their lifetime.

How ironic that the global slave trade was basically built around sugar, and to a lesser degree, so was its rotten cousin, alcohol (alcohol is rotten sugar). It's as if sugar and slavery go hand in hand, and always have done.

What other problems does it cause? It's when our blood sugar levels crash that drugs become an overwhelming temptation. Why? Because they raise our blood sugar, just like sugar does. Sugar leads to stimulant (drug) addiction for the vast majority of people.

What else? Sugar makes a perfect food for pathogenic micro organisms, which are organisms which mean us harm, including yeasts, fungi, moulds, bacteria and viruses. A cancer cell consumes four times as much sugar as a normal cell. These organisms, once encouraged with food, like leaving out food for rats, will start to cause havoc to all our bodily systems.

Another problem with sugar consumption is this: your liver and pancreas, which are in charge of managing your sugar levels, may go overboard and make you hypoglycaemic, or collapse entirely, causing type 2 diabetes.

Metabolising these sugars leaves an acidic residue, which our kidneys struggle to neutralise, and when the kidneys are weak that leaves us feeling anxious, stressed and exhausted. Do you see how this comes full circle?

Believe me when I say I'm only scratching the surface with the problems that sugar consumption causes. Two excellent books that go into detail about the problems are **Sugar Blues** and **Rainbow Green Live Food Cuisine** (see Resources section), the latter being particularly useful as it offers a practical alternative to a sugar-based diet.

Common Forms

A sugar, under this definition, is any simple carbohydrate. Even so-called complex carbohydrates, for instance bread or potatoes, become simple carbohydrates during the process of cooking. A baked potato actually causes more of a blood sugar spike than table sugar.

The Glycaemic Index is a method used by diabetics to measure their blood glucose response to foods. However, it can be misleading as it doesn't take into account how much of these foods are actually eaten.

Here is a partial list of sugary foods:

Anything containing flour of any kind

Cooked potatoes and carrots

Anything containing sugar, glucose syrup, high fructose corn syrup, corn starch, starch, maltose, dextrose, sucrose, lactose or maltodextrin should ideally be avoided as if it were contaminated with plague.

Corn, rice, wheat, rye, barley or anything containing these grains in any form

Any form of alcohol

Sweet fruits like banana, pineapple, dates or melons.

Even fruit, and whole grains?

Yes, even these contribute to the problem once you're on the sugar downward spiral. They can be reintroduced over time once the addiction is truly over. Grains have never been optimal foods for humans though: we started eating them because they're an easy way to feed large populations in big cities.

Natural fruits, which haven't been hybridised to be excessively sweet, are healthy once the habit is kicked. You can tell if a fruit is hybridised because it will have few or no seeds.

Caution

Be very wary indeed of anything marketing itself as sugar-free: usually the sweetener they use is even more dangerous and detrimental to health then sugar. Check the ingredients label and if you see anything where you don't know exactly what it is, don't touch it. **(see Processed Foods)**

Also, don't throw out the baby with the bathwater. Some sugars are essential to our health: these are known as polysaccharides. They tend to be bitter rather than sweet in taste. You find large quantities of these in fresh aloe vera, sea vegetables, goji berries, bee pollen and the medicinal mushrooms like shitake and reishi.

Cooked Fats

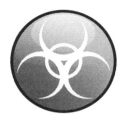

Description

The damaging effect of cooking fats has already been dealt with in the essential fats section earlier.

It's generally best not to eat cooked fat, with the exceptions of saturated fat – basically animal fat – and coconut oil. There fats are okay to heat. This isn't ideal, but they cope with being heated far better than most plant-based fats.

In order to reach true health it's ideal to not eat cooked vegetable fat, with the exception of coconut oil. If you are going to eat cooked fat, you're actually better off cooking with butter or lard than you are with sunflower oil or margarine. Margarine should be especially avoided at all costs, whatever the advertisers say. It's not good for your heart or any other part of your body. It's a highly profitable poison.

If you like cooked fatty, greasy food (like a fry up), cook with animal fats if you eat those, or, if you're a vegan, cook with coconut butter. Ideally go for coconut butter anyway, because it's probably the best source of fat to cook with out of all of them.

Common Forms

Avoid, as if your life depended on it (it does):

Fried food

Deep fried food

Ready meals

Baked food

Stir-fried food

Almost any food that comes out of a packet

Margarine

Junk food

Take away food

Restaurant food.

Vegetable oil almost always means cooked soya oil: probably the worst of the worst. Any oil you buy that doesn't emphasise that it's unheated and cold pressed.

Am I saying you can never have a roast dinner again? No, just that you should make it yourself, or it should be made by someone else who you can trust not to use poisonous cooked vegetable oils.

Recommended Action

Make a resolution to yourself that you'll eat abundantly of the healthy fat sources recommended in the Essential Fats section. When you do this the temptation to eat poisonous fats will decrease significantly.

Your body craves and loves fat because it needs it. You just need to refine its tastes by getting it used to the really good stuff.

Caution

Cooked vegetable oils are in almost all pre-prepared food. Assume it's there until proven otherwise. If you're eating out, make a big deal about being on a no fat diet and see what they can find that suits your needs. Then when you're home you can have a delicious high fat meal with healthy, raw fats to make up for it.

High Protein Diets

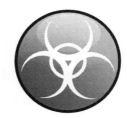

Description

The most famous of these is probably the Atkins diet. Some people do get some benefit from this approach, probably because it emphasises very strictly not having sugar, which can do you the world of good.

Bodybuilders and people who go to the gym are also guilty of making the mistake of eating excessive protein, although it often takes a while before they notice the symptoms as they're strong and healthy in other ways. The manifestation of problems with this kind of diet are inevitable though, eventually.

What we're focusing on right now is exhaustion, and exhaustion is basically a result of depleted kidneys. One of the main things that depletes the kidneys is a really high protein diet. Large amounts of animal protein especially, which includes dairy, puts a real strain on the kidneys.

If you're the sort of person who thinks that they need more protein, and are actually eating more protein to try to be healthier, all I can say is stop! Don't do it.

You have probably been endlessly told that you need more protein, especially if you're vegetarian or in the fitness world.

Yet all the research actually shows you that most people eat too much protein.

This myth we're fed telling us: "you need more protein; you need a high protein diet" is simply not true. It's similar to the lie we were told that somehow hydrogenated fats, in the form of margarine, were healthier than butter. It's the invention of a certain industry trying to sell a certain product, but it's not true.

If you believe that a high protein diet is good for you, maybe because you want to put on muscles and you've had that deeply ingrained, that's fine. These are only suggestions. But ideally, reduce protein in your diet as much as you can for the months you're doing this program, to give your body, and particularly your kidneys, a chance to recover.

Recommended Action

If you are really worried about protein, realise that the best sources of protein are green algaes like spirulina, chlorella and blue green algae. These green algaes are the highest source of protein known to man: they are around 60% protein by weight. In comparison to that the highest protein-containing animal foods, like fish, cheese, beef and chicken, are about 20%-30% protein at the most.

These far superior proteins found in algaes are easier to absorb, packed full of nutrition, and don't cause the same strain to the kidneys that animal proteins do.

Include them in your diet every day to be certain you're getting sufficient levels of the right, high quality protein.

Common Forms

Protein shakes

Protein bars

Meat

Fish

Eggs

Cheese

Soya

Nuts

Seeds

All of these, with the exception of nuts and seeds, would ideally be avoided. The worst of all is probably soya. Do not, in any circumstances, eat this incredibly harmful thyroid-suppressing substance as a health food. You're definitely better off with a steak, or almost anything for that matter.

Caution

The point is: if there are some high protein animal foods that you really enjoy, then by all means enjoy yourself. But don't eat high protein meals for the sake of being healthy: the very thought should strike you as absurd!

You could compare it to men in the early part of the 20th century smoking because they believed it made them more 'manly'!

Processed Foods

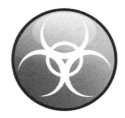

Description

Processed foods tend to be a conglomerate of every other dietary sin all rolled into one. They tend to be high in sugar and cooked fat, they often contain flavour enhancers that over- stimulate your central nervous system, and they even sometimes contain high quantities of animal protein.

But there's more! They tend to be devoid of any real nutrition, they're not fresh, and they contain an absolute multitude of toxic chemicals in the form of additives, colourings, flavour enhancers, preservatives, thickeners and emulsifiers.

There's a simple rule for any food you buy. Look at the ingredients label at the back carefully. If it contains anything you know is bad for you, as already listed, then don't buy it. If it contains anything that you don't even know what it is, don't buy it. You wouldn't put software you don't know onto your computer and you wouldn't put any old random liquid into the fuel tank of your car, so why play such a risky game with your own body?

Recommended Action

You'll notice, if you're willing to try this as an experiment, that this leaves almost no processed food you can eat.... which is very much the point. Raw organic superfood is close to ideal food, but you may well not be at that point yet.

So start on the road to an optimal diet with this simple step: avoid all processed foods entirely. There's always an alternative. The alternative might not be great either, but it will still be better, as processed food really is the lowest of the low. Just say no.

Common Forms

    All ready meals

    All fast food

    All junk food

    Anything advertised on TV

    Anything in a packet

    Anything you wouldn't know how to make from scratch yourself

    Anything with a long shelf life

    Anything containing an ingredient you don't recognise

Caution

Processed foods often contain many chemicals designed to

make them addictive. You may find yourself craving them, having withdrawal symptoms, feeling like nothing else is anywhere near as satisfying as.....

This is all standard drug withdrawal stuff, and will pass with time if you're persistent. Notice just how innocuous an addiction to these processed foods were, and then celebrate your freedom as soon as you feel the cravings start to subside..... you're free!

Sleep Deprivation

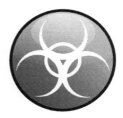

Description

Now, this would appear to be a really obvious point for an easy exhaustion cure: ideally don't deprive yourself of sleep! I know it sounds obvious – really going back to basics –but actually very few people, especially exhausted people, follow this simple bit of advice.

A lot of people act as if they think there's something clever, brave or heroic about not sleeping. If this sounds like you, let me be clear: there is nothing clever about it. You simply need to sleep. People need to sleep; people need to rest and recuperate.

What is sleep deprivation? The ideal amount of sleep you can have varies so much among people and their specific life situations. In fact, you may well need more one night than you did the night before. If you follow all the steps in this program you will ultimately need less sleep overall. However, sleep is still a healthy and necessary part of life.

Before the mass proliferation of the electric light bulb, people slept an average of nine hours a night. They also went to bed earlier, around the time it got dark. Now we sleep around six hours on average, and tend to go to bed after midnight. With this one simple statistic, the epidemic of exhaustion and all the health problems stemming from it could be explained.

Of course, once you are exhausted, sleep on its own isn't going to be enough to heal you. You've probably tried this and discovered it already. It is crucial, though, to be aware of the importance of the role of sleep in your life, and to remember this: when you are experiencing benefits as a result of doing this program, which you will be, don't start depriving yourself of sleep as you feel more energised. Allow yourself to sleep.

Common Forms

Ideally this section would have been earlier in this program as a must-do step, but I'm aware that some people just don't have the luxury of adequate sleep and I didn't want to exclude them from the program. It is possible to get real results with the program even if you deprive yourself of sleep, but it is more of an uphill journey.

The most common reasons people have for not sleeping enough are that they have a new baby or a busy job, or they have difficulty getting to sleep or staying asleep.

The latter two problems are addressed by this program, and you will find it easier to get to sleep and stay asleep as you follow all the steps.

If, however, your cause of sleep deprivation is outside of you, like a screaming baby, there's not a lot you can do about this. One observation I will make though: I've found that often people who have busy lives and claim that's the reason they are exhausted and sleep deprived spend a lot of time 'winding down' at the end of the day: time which would be more productively spent resting or sleeping.

They spend their time watching TV, or flicking through the internet. They usually say that if they did go to bed, they wouldn't be able to sleep. If this sounds like you, I urge you to increase the amount of the Taoist tonic herbs that cool the heart, like the Serenity blend. You have these in the evening and they help you to actually go to sleep as soon as there's an opportunity, rather than needing hours of staring at a screen to get you there.

Recommended Action

Don't try to force yourself to sleep long hours either. But, for instance, if as a result of using a grounding sheet, you feel like you don't want to get out of bed, and if you can avoid getting out of bed, then don't get out. Try and sleep for as long as you can, whenever you can. Never, ever think there's something big, clever or strong about depriving yourself of sleep.

Remember

Remember that all the recommendations in the bonus section are just that: recommendations. If you choose to carry on smoking, drinking coffee, eating cooked fat, depriving yourself of sleep, eating junk food and gorging on sugar, that's not going to exclude you from success in this program – although it may slow your progress down somewhat.

As long as you do all the other steps in this program, stick to them and do them for an absolute minimum of one month, preferably for three months, and ideally for a year, **you will get**

results: you will completely overcome your exhaustion, not just temporarily, not just for now, not until next time, but forever.

FINAL THOUGHTS

Keep It Simple

You've learned a hell of a lot during this program, and I hope much of it was enlightening, interesting and entertaining. But that's not what this book is for.

This is a call to action, pure and simple.

It's my fervent wish that I haven't overloaded you with information, but have just provided you with enough to prepare and inspire you to act.

Don't overcomplicate things. This cure is really very simple. You drink your kidney and heart tonic tea every day, or take your tonic herb tablets; you need to eat and drink some greens every day; eat your superfoods every day; take some supplements every day; you need to sleep on a grounding sheet; you need to get an early night on a less than full stomach whenever you can and you need to *breathe*.

That's it!

This is a program that's truly doable for anyone and everyone.

You can do it!

All the resources you need – like what to get, where from, when to do it and how much – are coming up in the last section of this book. Go for it! Start now, while it's fresh in your mind.

Get Leverage

How do you make sure you consistently follow through with this program so that your success is guaranteed? There are many different techniques for this, and if this is an area you struggle with, I highly suggest you seek out the work of a man called Anthony Robbins to show you how to motivate yourself.

You really do need to formulate a plan, not just for what you're going to do, which is what this program consists of, but also how you're going to make yourself do it consistently.

If you have someone else in your life who is more organised than you, who tends to be a nurturing person, who is highly invested in you getting better and who is willing and able to help with this program, then great. Share it with them and discuss what they can do to assist you.

Make a firm plan and stick to it. Don't let them derail you with what they think you should do: they're probably not health experts, because if they were you would have gone to them for advice in the first place.

If you can afford it, it's a fantastic idea to get some support from a coach, whose job it is to make sure you follow through on your goals by whatever means necessary.

A paid coach tends to be preferable to enrolling family or friends, because the sad fact is that most people have a lot invested in you staying as you are (they like/love you as you are, after all), while a coach's income depends on getting you to reach your goals.

However, if professional coaching isn't an option for you, there is a way to recruit a friend to help which is devastatingly effective. For this you'll need to find someone who can be your accountability partner.

The main qualities a person needs to be suitable for this are that they're trustworthy, they can tell if you're lying to them and they do what they say. You're going to make a little agreement with them.

Write a cheque to them, for an amount that you could just about afford to lose, but that it would pain you to do so. Something like a week's earnings should be sufficient unless you have a lot of savings, in which case more would be appropriate.

Next, get them to make this promise to you: if you don't follow the steps you've decided you'll do in this course every day, without fail, then they must cash that cheque and do what they like with the money.

Can you see how this could be a really good motivational tool to make sure you really stick to what you've set out to do? If not, increase the amount of money you'll lose until you see it.

This technique works beautifully. Your accountability partner is motivated to check up on you and see if you've stuck with your decision as it's easy money for them if you haven't. For you, so long as you stick with the program, you've just arranged free coaching, and you have powerful leverage on yourself to stick with it.

If the loss of money just doesn't move you, how about the

social pressure of looking like a failure in front of everyone you know, especially everyone who you look up to or whose opinion you care a lot about?

To use this powerful leverage tool, simply make an announcement. Tell everyone you know, especially all those whose opinions you value, what you are going to do, how long you'll do it for and why you're doing it. Ask them to encourage you by promising to taunt, tease and harass you if you give up.

Most people will readily agree to this. It's human nature: if you ask people to help you improve yourself, they tend to be underwhelmed at best. But if you set things up as a competition, people love to join in.

The important thing is this: set things up so success is inevitable and failure is not an option. Most people prepare for failure, and then get what they prepared for. Prepare for success: make failure seem so unbearable that you'll do whatever it takes to avoid it. Get creative: if loss of money or pride doesn't concern you as much as it does most people, what are you most afraid to lose? Put that thing on the line and success is guaranteed.

You could also take a 'before' photograph now, so you can track how much better you look as you progress with the program.

Remember that you have a very special destiny – an important part to play in this world – and that the only thing stopping you from doing that thing to your full potential is a lack of energy.

Believe in yourself. Believe in your capacity, and that you are worth it.

Whatever mistakes you may have made, whatever painful thing may have happened, it's time to start again, and your new life starts now.

Your Destiny awaits you!

Reassess Your Health

Now you've completed The Easy Exhaustion Cure for Workaholics and Overachievers, how much better are you? Check yourself on the questionnaire below, then compare your score to the original scores on page 21

The Easy Exhaustion Cure Questionnaire

Score the questionnaire as follows:

    0 for rarely or never

    1 for sometimes

    2 for frequently or always

1. Do you still feel tired 30 minutes after waking up?

2. Do you need a stimulant like tea, coffee or a cigarette to get started in the morning?

3. Do you need a stimulant like tea, coffee or a cigarette to keep you going throughout the day?

4. Do you crave sweet foods?

5. Do you crave starchy foods like bread, pasta, potatoes and crisps?

6. Do you feel like you need an alcoholic drink by the end of the day?

7. Are you overweight and do you have great trouble losing weight, despite dieting?

8. Do you have frequent slumps of energy?

9. Do they happen especially after meals?

10. Do you have mood swings?

11. Do you have difficulty concentrating?

12. Do you struggle to get out of bed in the morning?

13. Do you use the snooze button on your alarm in the morning?

14. Does your memory fail you for things which you consider important?

15. Does your sex drive feel lower than it was?

16. Do you tend to get overwhelmed easily?

17. Do you find it a struggle to adapt to changes in circumstances in life?

18. Does life seem to be moving too fast?

19. Do you feel your life is frequently immersed in some kind of drama?

20. Do you get dizzy, tired or irritable if you go for longer than 5 hours without eating something or taking a stimulant like tea, coffee or a cigarette?

21. Do you feel like you're ageing prematurely?

22. Do you frequently feel frustrated?

23. Do you frequently feel tired throughout the day?

24. Do you feel like no matter what you do it's never enough?

25. Have you had more than two colds or infections in the last two years?

26. Do you have dark circles under your eyes?

27. Do you feel more tired after exercise or exertion?

28. Do infections tend to linger?

29. Do you suffer from any inflammatory conditions like eczema or asthma?

30. Do you have any fungal conditions?

31. Do you become anxious easily?

32. Do you find yourself getting angry or annoyed over little things?

33. Do you feel a lack of motivation?

34. Do you have problems getting to sleep?

35. Do you have problems staying asleep?

Add up your total score _____ out of 70

Your Score Before _____

Your Score Now _____

Your Percentage Improvement (Before/Now x 100)

= % improvement _____

If you scored more than 30% improvement:

Congratulations! You obviously followed through on most, if not all of the recommendations in the program, and you're reaping the benefits. Keep at it as much as you can and things can only get better from here. You're on the right track now: you're off the cycle of energy depletion and on the path to energy abundance, if you're not already there. Keep going with these great new habits you've built and the world is your oyster.

If you scored between 15 and 30% improvement:

You're on the way, heading in the right direction. Perhaps you would benefit from incorporating more of the recommendations of this program, especially the recommendations in the bonus sections. You may find that it will take longer for you to get the full results of this program, but they will come. So stick with it, and do everything you can to move up to the next level in terms of your commitment to the recommendations given here.

If you scored less than 15% improvement:

I'm guessing that either you haven't followed the steps of this program in the way that they're described, or you were already extremely healthy. If you didn't really follow through on all the steps described, then now is the time to do it. Start again, see the first time as a practice run, and really go for it this time! Everything else was just preparation.

If you really did implement all the changes recommended for the full period of time, please contact me at <u>elwin@easyexhaustioncure.com</u> and I'll give you your money back. Your situation is probably very severe and you will almost certainly need a health expert to create a program tailored to your own unique situation. If that's the case please contact me and I promise I'll do my best to help.

ADDITIONAL INFORMATION AND RESOURCES

SHOPPING LIST

Below is a general list of many of the bare essentials, which you shouldn't run out of during the course of this program, to put on your shopping list. Remember to always buy organic wherever possible, i.e. unless it's not in stock.

While I've suggested that you get your fresh produce at a local shop, getting them direct from the farmers' market will be even better.

I've only included items here which are directly recommended in the program: other healthy options I'll leave up to your own taste and discretion.

Where appropriate I'll recommend a good brand or source. Where no recommendation is made, assume that quality is generally good, especially if you stick to buying from the retailers in the **Product Resources** section.

From Your Local Spring
- Fresh spring water

From Your Regular Shop or Supermarket
- Celery
- Cucumber
- Green leaves, like spinach, watercress, lettuce and fresh herbs
- Green vegetables
- Lemons
- Oysters
- Spring water

From Your Health Food Store or Online

- AFA blue green algae, like E3 Live or Elixir Of The Lake
- Brazil nuts
- Celtic sea salt, damp and grey
- Coconut oil, virgin cold pressed
- Flax oil, cold pressed
- Hemp oil, cold pressed
- Kelp powder, like Starwest Botanicals
- Pregnenolone, from Source Naturals
- Pumpkin seeds
- Sunflower seeds

Generally Available Online Only

- Angstrom mineral supplements e.g. zinc, Mineralife
- Green superfood powder blend like Vitamineral Green or Lion Heart Supergreens
- Grounding sheet, from Earth FX
- Krill oil, from Now Foods
- Healthforce Nutritionals Truly Natural Vitmain C or other or other food extract vitamin C supplement
- Magnesium oil, from Mineralife
- Marine phytoplankton, from Oceans Alive
- Orgono Living Silica or Horsetail herb, from Mountain Rose Herbs
- Rejuvenate Tonic Herbal Tea Blend
- Schizandra, from Lion Heart Herbs or Mountain Rose Herbs
- Serenity Tonic Herbal Tea blend from Lion Heart Herbs

Daily Schedule

'Dear diary, today I had my healthiest day ever...'

These daily schedules can be adapted to meet your own unique requirements. They assume that you are following the recommendations of this course exactly. Where no dose is given, follow the manufacturer's instructions. These are guidelines only: adapt them to your own tolerance level.

Starting Dosages

These recommendations apply to week one of the course: days one to seven.

On waking

500ml or 1 pint of spring water with a pinch of celtic sea salt and/or

Rehydrate and a squeeze of lemon juice added.

Angstrom mineral supplements: zinc and others

Apply magnesium oil

Daily multiple

Pregnenolone 1x 25mg tablet

Before breakfast

500ml or 1 pint of green juice

Breathing exercise, 5 minutes (optional but highly encouraged)

Breakfast

One green superfood smoothie with anything else you like, bearing in mind the recommendations in the **Ideally Don't** section.

With breakfast

Vitamin C, 4x 500mg plant extract tablet

Krill oil, 1x 500mg tablet

Mid-morning snack

½ teaspoon of AFA blue green algae in 500ml spring water and/or 5 drops of marine phytoplankton

Apply magnesium oil

Before lunch

Breathing exercise, 5 minutes (optional but highly encouraged)

Lunch

Whatever you like, bearing in mind the suggestions in the **Ideally don't** section

Fill half of your plate with green leaves

Pour on cold-pressed seed oil and sprinkle on raw salt

During the day

Kidney tonic tea made with 15g of herbs or 4x 500mg tablets

Schizandra tonic tea made with 15g of schizandra or 4x 500mg tablets, if not already contained in kidney tonic herbs

At least another 1000ml or 2 pints of spring water with a pinch of salt and/or Rehydrate added

Apply magnesium oil

Afternoon snack

Ideally nothing, but if required, a handful of raw seeds and brazil nuts with goji berries

Before dinner

Breathing exercise, 5 minutes (optional but highly encouraged)

Dinner

Whatever you like, bearing in mind the suggestions in the **Ideally don't** section

Fill half of your plate with green leaves

Pour on cold-pressed seed oil and sprinkle on raw salt

With dinner

Krill oil, 1x 500mg

Before bed

Heart tonic tea made with 15g of herbs, or 4x 500mg tablets

Apply magnesium oil

Sleep

On grounding sheet

By 10pm

In a dark, ventilated room

For as long as you feel the need

Intermediate Dosages

These recommendations apply to week two of the program, days eight to fourteen.

On waking

750ml or 1 ½ pints of spring water with a pinch of Celtic sea salt and/or Rehydrate and a squeeze of lemon juice added.

Angstrom mineral supplements: zinc and others

Apply magnesium oil

Daily multiple

Pregnenolone 1x 25mg tablet

Before breakfast

Breathing exercise, 10 minutes (optional but highly encouraged)

750ml or 1 ½ pints of green juice

Breakfast

One green superfood smoothie with anything else you like, bearing in mind the recommendations in the **Ideally Don't** section

With breakfast

Vitamin C, 4x 500mg plant extract tablet

Krill oil, 1x 500mg tablet

Mid-morning snack

1 teaspoon of AFA blue green algae in 500ml spring water and/or

15 drops of marine phytoplankton

Apply magnesium oil

Before lunch

Breathing exercise, 5 minutes (optional but highly encouraged)

Lunch

Whatever you like, bearing in mind the suggestions in the **Ideally don't** section

Fill half of your plate with green leaves

Pour on cold-pressed seed oil and sprinkle on raw salt

With lunch

Vitamin C, 4x 500mg plant extract tablet

Krill oil, 1x 500mg tablet

During the day

Kidney tonic tea made with 30g of herbs or 8x 500mg tablets

Schizandra tonic tea made with 30g of schizandra or 8x 500mg tablets, if not already contained in kidney tonic herbs

At least another 1000ml or 2 pints of spring water with a pinch of salt and/or Rehydrate added

Apply magnesium oil

Afternoon snack

Ideally nothing, but if required, a handful of raw seeds and brazil nuts with goji berries

Before dinner

Breathing exercise, 5 minutes (optional but highly encouraged)

Dinner

Whatever you like, bearing in mind the suggestions in the **Ideally don't** section

Fill half of your plate with green leaves

Pour on cold-pressed seed oil and sprinkle on raw salt

With dinner

Krill oil, 1x 500mg

Before bed

Heart Tonic Tea made with 30g of herbs, or 8x 500mg tablets

Apply magnesium oil

Sleep

On grounding sheet

By 10pm

In a dark, ventilated room

For as long as you feel the need

Full Dosages

These recommendations apply to weeks three to twelve of the program – days fourteen to ninety – and beyond, ideally.

On waking

1000ml or 2 pints of spring water with a pinch of Celtic sea salt and/or Rehydrate and a squeeze of lemon juice added. More if desired

Angstrom mineral supplements: zinc and others

Apply magnesium oil

Daily multiple

Orgono Living Silica

Pregnenolone 1x 50mg tablet

Before breakfast

Breathing exercise, 15 minutes (optional but highly encouraged)

1000ml or 2 pints of green juice, more if desired.

Breakfast

One green superfood smoothie with anything else you like, bearing in mind the recommendations in the **Ideally Don't** section

With breakfast

Vitamin C, 4x 500mg plant extract tablet

Krill oil, 2x 500mg tablet

Mid-morning snack

1 teaspoon of AFA blue green algae in 500ml spring water and/or

15 drops of marine phytoplankton

Apply magnesium oil

Before lunch

Breathing exercise, 10 minutes (optional but highly encouraged)

Lunch

Whatever you like, bearing in mind the suggestions in the **Ideally don't** section

Fill half of your plate with green leaves

Pour on cold-pressed seed oil and sprinkle on raw salt

With lunch

Vitamin C, 4x 500mg plant extract tablet

Krill oil, 1x 500mg tablet

During the day

Kidney tonic tea made with 60g of herbs or 12x 500mg tablets, more if desired

Schizandra tonic tea made with 60g of schizandra or 12x 500mg tablets, if not already contained in kidney tonic herbs. More if desired

At least another 1000ml or 2 pints of spring water with a pinch of salt added and/or Rehydrate , ideally a lot more

15 drops or more of marine phytoplankton throughout the day

Apply magnesium oil

Afternoon snack

Ideally nothing, but if required, a handful of raw seeds and brazil nuts with goji berries

Before dinner

Breathing exercise, 10 minutes (optional but highly encouraged)

Dinner

Whatever you like, bearing in mind the suggestions in the **Ideally don't** section

Fill half of your plate with green leaves

Pour on cold-pressed seed oil and sprinkle on raw salt

With dinner

Krill oil, 1x 500mg

Vitamin C, 4x 500mg plant extract tablet

Before bed

Heart tonic tea made with 30g of herbs, or 8x 500mg tablets

Apply magnesium oil

Sleep

On grounding sheet

By 10pm whenever possible

In a dark, ventilated room

For as long as you feel the need

Maintenance Dosages

These are, again, only recommendations. But once you've finished the program, because you feel better than ever, you'll probably be reluctant to stop these things which have transformed your life so radically – and rightly so.

Follow these recommendations to consolidate the gains you've made, and, if you're ready for the next level, keep your eye out for the next instalment from Lion Heart Solutions...

On waking

750ml or 1 ½ pints of spring water with a pinch of Celtic sea salt and a squeeze of lemon juice added.

Angstrom mineral supplements: zinc and others

Apply magnesium oil

Before Breakfast

Breathing exercise, 10 minutes (optional but highly encouraged)

750ml or 1 ½ pints of green juice

Breakfast

One green superfood smoothie with anything else you like, bearing in mind the recommendations in the **Ideally Don't** section

With breakfast

Vitamin C, 4x 500mg plant extract tablet

Krill oil, 1x 500mg tablet

Mid-morning snack

1 teaspoon of AFA blue green algae in 500ml spring water and/or

15 drops of marine phytoplankton

Before lunch

Breathing exercise, 10 minutes (optional but highly encouraged)

Lunch

Whatever you like, bearing in mind the suggestions in the **Ideally don't** section

Fill half of your plate with green leaves

Pour on cold-pressed seed oil and sprinkle on raw salt

During the day

Kidney tonic tea made with 30g of herbs or 8x 500mg tablets

At least another 1000ml or 2 pints of spring water with a pinch of salt added

Afternoon snack

Ideally nothing, but if required, a handful of raw seeds and brazil nuts with goji berries

Before dinner

Breathing exercise, 10 minutes (optional but highly encouraged)

Dinner

Whatever you like, bearing in mind the suggestions in the **Ideally don't** section

Fill half of your plate with green leaves

Pour on cold- pressed seed oil and sprinkle on raw salt

With dinner

Krill oil, 1x 500mg

Sleep

On grounding sheet

By 10pm

In a dark, ventilated room

For as long as you feel the need

Additional Dietary Recommendations

The following dietary recommendations are, of course, suggestions only, but they're very helpful ones that you'll experience significant benefit from heeding:

Eat lightly of heavy, unhealthy foods.

Eat abundantly of light, healthy foods.

Chew your food thoroughly.

Eat earlier in the day.

Never skip breakfast.

Don't drink for an hour or two after your food, and definitely not during your meal, unless it's Kombucha or carbonated spring water with lemon.

Eat a large percentage of high water content food, basically fresh, raw fruits and vegetables.

Eat a majority of plant food.

Eat a significant amount of green food.

Eat a diet where ideally 80% of what you eat is alkaline-forming.

Eat your plant food raw, or as raw as possible,

unless you find it hard to digest that way.

What you don't eat raw, ideally eat steamed, boiled or in soups and stews. Baking, roasting, frying, grilling, deep frying etc. is particularly damaging to foods. Ideally prepare in a way in which the water content is preserved.

Eat as much nutritionally dense food as possible. This especially means superfoods, as well as the ones listed earlier try: goji berries, seaweeds, bee pollen, raw chocolate, maca, suma, carob, aloe vera, young coconuts and coconut butter, acai, noni, hempseeds, incan berries, ashwagandha, chaga, sacha jargon and fresh vanilla. If you don't know what to do with any of them, try throwing them all in a blender and making a 'superfood smoothie.' Experiment, and find the ones you love!

Add unpasteurised cultured food to your diet as much as possible. Raw sauerkraut is the most well-known and widely available version of this.

Unless you have severe blood sugar issues, eat infrequently and give your digestion a chance to relax. Just two meals a day is ideal, but you may have to build up to this. Remember that despite the modern myths, which are a hangover from the times when food really was scarce, you're far more likely to be harmed by an excess of food than a lack, especially as your nutritional needs are being met with this program.

Don't be afraid of fatty foods so long as they're unheated, including before you bought them. Only cooked fat is unhealthy and makes you fat.

Additional Supplement Recommendations

In addition to all the supplements listed in this program, these supplements, while not targeted to exhaustion specifically, are universally beneficial for those seeking optimum health.

Astaxanthin and Resveratol are excellent antioxidants with many well-researched and proven health benefits. NOW does a good version of both, 4mg and 200mg being good doses respectively.

Betaine HCL is especially useful for those with a weak digestion. NOW is a great brand; 650mg with every meal is a great dose.

Indium Sulphate helps to absorb trace minerals far better. Indiumase is great brand; 1-2 drops a day is plenty.

Medicinal Mushroom Blend, to educate your immune system. Source Naturals Immune Defence is an excellent 16-mushroom blend, the more the better.

Melatonin can be a life-saver for those who can't get to sleep. However, for many reasons, not least because we quickly build up a tolerance and it stops working, habitual use is not recommended. It's handy to have around for special occasions though. 3mg is a good dose; NOW do a great sublingual fast-action tablet form.

Methylcobalamin is a powerful form of vitamin B12. Jarrow do a great 100mcg formula.

MSM *is excellent for hair, skin, nails, lungs, the liver, any inflammation or allergic reaction and joint pain. Start at 1-2g a day, building up slowly over several months to 10-20g a day. Source Naturals do a good brand, but it's all pretty much the same.*

Probiotics *for intestinal health. Nature's Best are excellent quality.*

Vitamin D3 *is one of the most important and depleted vitamins in the body. Doses of around 5000iu are effective in most cases; NOW do a great brand, as does Dr Mercola.*

Vitamin K2 *is another overlooked but vital vitamin; NOW do a great one, 50mcg is a good dose.*

Zeolites *are a fantastic way to detoxify anything out of your body, gently. Zeoforce is an excellent brand, the more the better.*

Fulvic Acid *is an excellent addition to water to make it more hydrating, and also to bring nutrients into the body and get toxins out. Mineralife do a great quality version*

Additional Practice Recommendations

These practices would all be excellent to incorporate into your life, but were generally not included in the main part of the program as they don't quite come under the classification of easy.

Colonic Hydrotherapy

If ever you feel under the weather in any way, please do me a favour: don't reach for some kind of drug or supplement to suppress the symptoms. Instead, go and have a colonic. This is especially vital during this program. Any time you have an illness of any kind, the root cause is always at least partially an excess of toxicity.

Usually, clearing the large intestine, the body's main exit route for this toxicity, resolves any symptoms you're having. This is true if you're being unhealthy, and the toxicity is building up, or if you're trying to be healthy, and therefore the toxicity is being released.

If ever I feel unwell in any way, I never think, "I must have caught something, I'm getting ill", I simply think, "my toxicity must be being released at a rate where my eliminative organs are getting overwhelmed and the toxicity is getting backed up: time to have colonic hydrotherapy."

You may disagree with my reasoning, but you can't argue with the result. I always feel better immediately, and so will you. Give it a try.

Chi Kung

This simply means 'energy cultivation', and comes down to becoming aware of, and then learning to direct and focus, your own energy, as well as connecting to the sources of energy around you. We've already discussed one of those sources, Planet Earth, which gives us grounding energy as scientists have recently verified.

What you then do with this energy is up to your own predilection, and there are various schools which have different goals in mind. Common uses for energy include becoming a great warrior, healer, athlete, scholar, lover or spiritual master.

Whatever your interest, cultivating energy can help you achieve it. This program has shown you how to do it with your diet and lifestyle: chi kung can show you how to cultivate energy using your will.

Information Resources

Here are a variety of information resources to find out more about everything introduced during this program:

Audio Learning

Anthony Robbins	Living Health
	The Body You Deserve
David Wolfe	All the information on thebestdayever.com
Shazzie	All the information on shazziesviproom.com

Books

A True Ott	Wellness Secrets for Life
Annie and David Jubb	Secrets of an Alkaline Body
Barbara Wren	Cellular Awakening
Clint Ober	Earthing
David Wolfe	The Sunfood Diet Success System
	Eating for Beauty
	Superfoods
Edward Howell	Enzyme Nutrition: The Food Enzyme Concept
Emil I Mondoa	Sugars That Heal
Gabriel Cousens	Rainbow Green Live Food Cuisine
Gillian McKeith	Miracle Superfood: Wild Blue Green Algae
John Robbins	Diet For a New America

Mantak Chia	Awaken Healing Energy Through The Tao
	Taoist Cosmic Healing
Masaru Emoto	The Hidden Message in Water
Mike Nash	Aggressive Health
Patrick Holford	The Optimum Nutrition Bible
Robert Young	Sick And Tired
	The PH Miracle Diet
Ron Teeguarden	The Ancient Wisdom of the Chinese Tonic Herbs
Sarma Melngailis	Living Raw Food
	Raw Food, Real World
Shazzie	Detox Your World
	Evie's Kitchen
Stu Mittleman	Slow Burn
Udo Erasmus	Fats and Oils

How-to Videos

Making Green Juice

http://www.lionheartherbs.com/index.php/how-to/how-to-make-the-best-easiest-green-juice-ever

Making Green Superfood Smoothie

http://www.lionheartherbs.com/index.php/how-to/how-to-make-a-green-smoothie

Making Taoist Tonic Tea

http://www.lionheartherbs.com/index.php/how-to/how-to-best-prepare-your-taoist-tonic-herbs

Magazines

Get Fresh

Passion

Websites

anthonyrobbins.com

thebestdayever.com

Earthing.net

gnosischocolate.com

philipmccluskey.com

Lionheartherbs.com

Oneluckyduck.com

Shazzie.com

Successultranow.com

Universal-tao.com

Product Resources

Listed here are the online retailers I highly recommend. They come in two categories:

Top quality retailers

These retailers only provide the best products. You can feel confident that anything you buy from them is of the highest quality. Their prices often reflect this, although not always:

- Detoxyourworld.com
- Dragonherbs.com
- Earthing.net
- Healthforcenutritionals.com
- gnosischocolate.com
- philipmccluskey.com
- Lionheartherbs.com
- Mineralifeonline.com
- Mountainroseherbs.com
- Oneluckyduck.com
- Starwestbotanicals.com

Mixed quality retailers

These retailers also sell a lot of high quality merchandise; otherwise they wouldn't appear on this list. However, they stock a lot of products of all quality levels and leave it up to their customers to decide what they want to invest in.

- Aggressivehealthshop.co.uk
- Highernature.co.uk
- Iherb.com

Best Retailers

In Europe:

My own site, www.lionheartherbs.com, sells pretty much everything you need to do this program, with the exception of grounding sheets, which you get from www.aggressivehealthshop.co.uk

All the products mentioned in this program are conveniently listed in the 'Easy Exhaustion Cure' category in www.lionheartherbs.com.

Initially, when this program first came out, the only things that

I was recommending and selling were the herbs mentioned. I'm recommending everything in here because I know it works, and because I use it myself, or have done.

However, I found the most common question I was getting by far wasn't what I was expecting. It was basically 'Where do I get this from?' and 'Isn't there somewhere I can get all this stuff from in one place?'

Two excellent questions – and I discovered there wasn't.

So I created it.

In the Americas:

You can obtain the herbal blends recommended in this program from:
www.lovingraw.com
www.oneluckyduck.com
www.gnosischocolate.com

You can find everything else you need from
www.mineralifeonline.com,
www.iherb.com and
www.longevitywarehouse.com.

The rest of the world:

Depending where you are, either of these two options may be most appropriate for you.

If other distributors become available in other parts of the world, I'll be sure to keep you updated.

About Lion Heart Solutions

Over 90% of the western world suffers from exhaustion, stress and/or anxiety at some point in their lives. Over 70% of people suffer from these conditions most of their lives.

Over 90% of the western world is addicted to refined sugars and stimulants like tea, coffee, tobacco, chocolate, alcohol, cocaine and caffeinated soft drinks.

These two figures are **most definitely related.**

The results of this chronic addiction to stimulants and sugar are severely detrimental to the individual, to society and to the world.

On an individual level, daily stimulant use leads to:

1. Physical weakness, as stimulants drain you of vital energy – leaving you open to pain, sickness and disease.

2. Mental depletion, as your central nervous system gets chronically over-stimulated – before long leaving you in a mental fog much of the time, struggling to focus or comprehend anything new.

3. Emotional turbulence: as your blood sugar levels destabilise, your average day becomes an emotional rollercoaster. This is exhausting and overwhelming, and feels intolerable without another hit of your stimulant of choice.

4. A loss of integrity caused by the internal conflict engendered by stimulant addiction: you sense deep down that your addiction doesn't ultimately serve you, or those around you, or the planet, yet you find it almost impossible to stop.

On a societal level, when you're stressed, exhausted and addicted, you're rarely living up to your highest potential, as this requires a significant amount of energy.

Even if you are living up to your highest potential by sheer willpower, if you're also stressed, exhausted and using stimulants, then you won't be living up to your highest potential for very long: you'll burn out and collapse.

Anyone not living up to their full potential for as long as they can is a terrible waste from society's point of view. Imagine all the good they could have done. What creative solutions might they have implemented to better us all, if only they'd had the energy to see it through?

Imagine a world where not only did people in more affluent countries have the opportunity to live up their full potential in theory, as they do now, but they actually had enough energy to really grasp and follow through on that potential. What sort of society would we live in? What sort of world would we create if we were free of energy depletion and addiction?

On a planetary level, the cost of the western world's stimulant use is exorbitant.

Currently over 25% of the world's agricultural resources are being used to grow stimulants and refined sugars. At the same time 40,000 children die every day of starvation.

My aims are that by 2030, the figure will be reduced to under 3% of our agricultural resources being used to grow stimulants and refined sugar, and that fewer than 40 children a day will die of starvation.

I understand that prohibition of any drug has never really worked, therefore the only way to achieve this figure is to:

> A) Educate people about stimulants and sugar: what they are, what they do and how they work.
>
> B) Offer a truly appealing and realistic alternative, teaching about economising the energy of the body: how to get more energy, how to stop it from being wasted, why this is so important, and what you can do with this energy if you have it.
>
> C) Offer that solution in a way that is compelling, simple and easy to use.

When people in the western world learn these distinctions about stimulants and sugar, and apply them to their lives, the results will be truly extraordinary.

Free of stimulant and sugar addiction, we will no longer waste energy: we will have it in abundance. This, combined with the relative comfort and freedom we enjoy in the western world, and the compassion naturally present in people – but sadly lacking in those who use drugs, including stimulants, to distract and numb themselves – will empower us.

We'll naturally use our abundant energy, compassion and freedom to create and implement solutions that will bring about abundance for everyone on Earth, so that ultimately no one has to struggle just to survive. Everyone will have their basic needs met for quality food, water, clothes and shelter, and everyone will have the opportunity to learn and develop themselves so they in turn can express their full potential and contribute to the world.

Demand for stimulants and sugar, mostly grown in the third world, will decrease, while simultaneously demand for superfoods and herbs will inevitably increase as people realise what an excellent alternative they are. Lion Heart Solutions is committed to helping provide education on all aspects of growing these new, healthier, more resource-efficient crops in place of sugar and stimulants.

This education will focus on growing these sustainable crops in a way which benefits the land, feeds and benefits the society they're grown in, and provides high quality nutrition for a new generation of consumers in the western world who will inevitably demand it.

Lion Heart Solutions is determined to make this change in the allocation of the world's resources by reducing exhaustion, and concurrently stimulant and refined sugar abuse, to less than 10% of the population in the western world from the +90% it's at now.

With this done, all our other goals will be achieved effortlessly. A new era of abundance, where everyone in the world's basic needs are met and where everyone has an opportunity to fulfil their potential, will dawn.

It has to. Mutually-assured destruction is the only other option. Our current way of life is not sustainable on any level: personal, societal and especially on a planetary level. We're all in this together, and the sooner we can replace our addictions with something better – something that elevates us rather than keeps us enslaved – the sooner we won't be able to avoid this simple truth any longer. This realisation is inevitable. The only question is: how painful is it going to be?

I believe the targets to be totally realistic, so long as the right information is presented to enough people in the right way – one which truly causes people to take action and make a change. This is my specialty.

If you are interested in supporting this happening, please contact me at elwin@easyexhaustioncure.com

ABOUT ELWIN ROBINSON

Elwin is a Tonic Herbalist, Nutritionist, Health Consultant, Author and Motivational Speaker.

Elwin is the founder of Lion Heart Herbs and Lion Heart Solutions, author of The Easy Exhaustion Cure and the forthcoming 'Raw Transformation' and 'Official Detox Guide' He's the creator of 'The Easy Exhaustion Cure' program, and the 'Complete Detox Course' an interactive and practical online course. He's a regular contributor to the magazines 'Get Fresh' and 'Passion'.

Elwin has worked with all kinds of clients to get results, several of whom are notable health practitioners and experts themselves, quickly getting a reputation for really helping people. He has spoken at many events throughout the world and led several health retreats.

Elwin specialises in helping people with low energy, stress, detoxification, blood sugar balance and removing opportunistic organisms. His approach is to strengthen and balance the body until health is inevitable.

Elwin won't truly rest until every person in the world has abundant energy with all the passion, love, strength, courage, enthusiasm, joy and clarity that this provides.

Elwin is utterly convinced that the Earth is a wonderfully abundant place, and that all that really needs to happen to make the whole human race activate their full potential and live in harmonious interdependence with each other, is that we just need to raise and hone our awareness to be aware of this abundance and start creating the world that all utopian dreamers have envisaged throughout the ages.

Elwin believes that the only way this transformation can come about is if every person has an abundance of energy at every level, at which point everything will start to fall into place for everyone, our boundless creativity will find solutions for every problem our lack of energy and subsequent lack of awareness has brought about, and we will use our vastly enhanced understanding to reach the stars and beyond.

Elwin is passionately dedicated to doing his part to make this transformation come about, through his practical contributions: step by step programs on how to reach a state of energetic abundance, as well as by example, through his own personal growth and self actualisation. Elwin is totally opposed to any hypocrisy, and firmly believes we need to be the change we wish to see in the world.

Elwin's approach focuses on simple, practical ways to maximise results in the most long term, effective way for life. He uses a combination of cutting edge scientific discoveries and ancient knowledge relevant to modern day life, to create the best systems for radical transformation in the areas of health, energy and vitality.

Elwin's passion for results and impeccability has led him to study a vast selection of systems and approaches for lasting health and energy transformation in order to find the most accurate and effective methods, it is this work that has led him to the creation of his business and products, bringing you the best of the best that is currently available.

Having battled health and energy problems throughout his early life this led him to this journey of discovery. He comes from a perspective of getting results and sharing the methods that have culminated in a total transformation of his life and the lives of his clients.

Elwin's no-nonsense, practical approach combined with his passion and vitality are a captivating combination that inspires and motivates people to achieve their potential for vibrant health, abundant energy and glowing wellbeing. This is not only a possibility, but a guarantee as a result of following his systems for success.

To work with Elwin one to one, contact him at elwin@easyexhaustioncurre.com to arrange a consultation.